Hearthwarming

Tried and True Recipes from Grandma's Kitchen

Janet C. Stocks

Opal Kingdom Press

Print ISBN: 978-1-952415-16-6

Cover by Melissa McShane

Photography by Carly Stocks

Contents

Foreword

I cannot remember a time that family life with Janet C. Stocks didn't revolve around being in the kitchen. As I am the oldest of her six children, I can confidently say that means her love of cooking and recipes goes back a very long time. In the kitchen, we made meals, shared secrets, talked about life and love and growing up.

If it wasn't enough to bless her own children's lives through food and eating together, Mom shared her skills with local church groups, and with enthusiastic 4-H clubs. When she went back to university, she took on adding an understanding of the food science that backed everything she knew by history and instinct. She quickly joined the faculty, teaching twelve years worth of college students. They didn't just learn how to MAKE food from Mom, they learned, like we had, how to love it. They learned about flavors. They learned about what golden brown and delicious looked like, and what perfect cake tops felt like. They learned that who you shared a meal with was just as important as what the meal was, and the sharing was about far more than just nutrition.

Which all leads me to this cookbook. Gathered here are recipes carried through all those years. These are the top shelf recipes that have never been far out of reach. These are the recipes that defined not only my life, but many others.

We can never say thank you enough for all the lessons learned. The only way we can try is to pass them on.

We love you, Mom.

Jana Brown on behalf of her siblings, many grateful students, and eaters

A note...

Some of these recipes call specifically for E-Z Gel® or ThickGel®. These are specialty starches developed by Janet in the mid 90s as she tried to solve some kitchen quandries like sauces that wouldn't hold in the fridge and cookies that dried out far too easily. They continue to be sold in local Utah stores and through the Cornaby's website, Cornaby's being the specialty food company that she co-owns with her brother. They are awesome products, and we stand behind them, however, because we know not everyone can easily lay hands on these products, we've adjusted recipes where we can to give alternatives for more commonly available starches and thickeners. There are a few exceptions where these products are absolutely required to make the recipe work and in those cases we've left it as is.

Appetizers and Beverages

Appetizers

Ham and Cheese Quiche

- 1 egg, well beaten
- 1 unbaked 9″ or 10″ pie crust
- 1 c. ham
- 1 c. cheese of your choice
- 4 eggs
- 1 c. milk
- ½ t. salt and ¼ t. pepper

Brush beaten egg over surface of unbaked pie crust. Bake at 375° for 10 minutes until golden brown. Remove from oven and layer ham and cheese on crust. Combine other ingredients, beating well with wire whisk. Pour over ingredients in baked crust and return to oven to bake an additional 40 - 50 minutes until filling is set and lightly browned.

Yield: 4-6 servings

Sausage and Cheese Strata

- 6 slices bread
- 1 ½ c. grated cheddar cheese
- 4 ounces mild sausage, browned and drained
- 2 T. chopped onion
- 3 eggs
- 1 ½ cups milk
- 1 t. salt
- ¼ t. pepper

Cube bread slices. Place half of the bread cubes in 9″ square baking dish or casserole. Layer with ¾ c. grated cheese and half of the browned sausage. Repeat with remaining bread cubes, cheese and sausage. Combine remaining ingredients and pour over bread layers. Cover with plastic wrap and refrigerate over night (or at least 4 hours). Bake at 325° about 1 hour until knife inserted in center comes out clean. Let stand 5 minutes before cutting.

Mushroom Strata: Prepare Sausage and Cheese Strata as directed, adding one half of a 10½-oz. can condensed cream of mushroom soup to egg mixture and reducing milk to 1 cup. Add one 4-oz. can sliced mushrooms.

Yield: 4 servings

Christmas Cheese Ball

- 3 (5 oz.) bottles Old English cheese spread
- 16 oz. cream cheese, softened
- 1 T. Worcestershire sauce
- 1 t. onion powder
- 1 c. shredded cheese
- 1 c. chopped nuts – opt

Cream ingredients, except nuts, together. Chill for about 2 hours. Divide in half and roll into logs or balls. Roll in chopped nuts and wrap in plastic wrap. Chill overnight to let flavors meld.

Yield: 2 medium or 3 small cheeseballs

Beverages

Orange Julius

- ½ c. milk
- ½ c. water
- ½ c. frozen orange juice concentrate
- ½ t. vanilla extract
- ¼ c. sugar or alternative sweetener
- 5-6 regular or 10 small ice cubes

Combine first 5 ingredients in blender container. Process until blended. Add ice cubes, one at a time, and blend until smooth. Serve.

Yield: 2 servings

Strawberry Julius

Make as Orange Julius replacing orange juice concentrate with 1/4 c. strawberry preserves and a handful of washed and stemmed fresh strawberries.

Yield: 2 servings

Banana Slush

- 1 12-oz. can frozen orange juice concentrate
- 1 12-oz can frozen lemonade concentrate
- 5 bananas, mashed fine

- 1 21-oz. can crushed pineapple
- 3 c. sugar
- 6 c. water
- 2 or 3 2-liter bottles lemon-lime soda

Combine first six ingredients. Pour into flat freezer-safe containers and freeze until firm. Remove mixture from freezer 20-30 minutes before breaking into chunks and serving with chilled soda.

Yield: 24 servings

Russian Tea

- 11 c. water
- 1 ¼ c. sugar
- 1 ½ cinnamon sticks
- 6 cloves
- 1 c. pineapple juice
- ½ c. lemon juice
- 6 oz orange juice concentrate

Bring to a boil the water, sugar, cinnamon, and cloves. Simmer for 15 minutes. Add the pineapple juice, lemon juice and orange juice concentrate. Serve hot or cold.

Yield: Enough to cure many

Fruit Smoothie

- ½ c. chopped frozen fruit or berries
- 1½ c. milk or alternative (almond, oat, etc.)
- ¼-½ c. sugar or alternative (to taste)
- 6-8 ice cubes

Combine fruit, milk, and sugar in blender container. Process until blended. Add ice cubes, one at a time. Blend until smooth. Serve. If desired, ½ c. yogurt or ice cream may be added for additional creaminess.

Yield: 2 servings

Salads and Dressings

Salads

Fresh Fruit Salad

- 1 (16 oz.) can fruit cocktail in light syrup or 100% juice
- 1 (20 oz.) can pineapple chunks in 100% juice
- 1 T. orange juice concentrate
- ½ t. vanilla
- 3 T. E-Z Gel®
- 2 c. sliced or diced fresh fruit (bananas, apples, strawberries, etc.)

Drain juice from fruit cocktail and pineapple chunks into a medium bowl (reserve fruit) and combine with orange juice concentrate, vanilla and cold water (if necessary) to make 1 cup. Gradually add E-Z Gel®, stirring with a wire whisk. Allow five minutes for salad to thicken. Add fresh fruit and reserved canned fruit and stir to coat with thickened dressing. Serve immediately or refrigerate. Store leftover dressing in the refrigerator for up to one week. **Fluffy Fruit Salad**: Prepare Fresh Fruit Salad as directed. Fold in 2 cups whipped cream just before serving.

Yield: 12 servings

Strawberry and Spinach Salad

Wash and trim 4 cups fresh spinach. Wash, hull, and slice 1 cup fresh strawberries. Combine and refrigerate.

Add ⅓ cup sugar, ¼ cup cider vinegar, ½ teaspoon dehydrated minced onion, ¼ teaspoon paprika, and ½ teaspoon Worcestershire sauce to blender container. Process for 30 seconds. Add ¼ cup oil, blending an additional 30 seconds. Stir in poppy seeds. Refrigerate. Pour over spinach and strawberry salad just before serving. For more variety and extra crunch sprinkle salad with a few pomegranate seeds and some candied walnuts or pecans.

Yield: 4-6 servings

Salad Dressings and Dips

Orange Blossom Dip

- 1 c. light sour cream
- 1 c. milk
- ½ c. sugar
- 4 T. orange juice concentrate, thawed
- ½ t. vanilla
- ¼ c. E-Z Gel® or 2 T. instant vanilla pudding

Stir sour cream until smooth. Add milk, sugar, orange juice concentrate and vanilla. Gradually add E-Z Gel®, stirring constantly with a wire whisk until smooth and creamy. Serve with fresh fruit: apples (unpeeled for color), bananas, pineapple, strawberries, grapes, etc.

Yield: 2 1/2 cups

Dilly Vegetable Dip

- 1 c. EACH sour cream and mayonnaise
- 1 T. chopped green onions
- 1 t. dill weed and 1 t. salt
- 1 t. lemon juice
- 1 t. parsley

Combine all ingredients. Chill. Serve with fresh vegetables.

Yield: 2 cups

Onion Dip

- 2 T. dehydrated minced onion
- ½ t. EACH garlic powder and onion powder
- 1 t. salt
- 1 t. low sodium beef bouillon granules OR beef soup base
- 2 T. E-Z Gel®
- ½ c. EACH light mayonnaise and light sour cream
- 1 c. buttermilk

Toast dehydrated onion in preheated oven at 400° for about 5 minutes. Cool. Combine with remaining dry ingredients. Combine mayonnaise and buttermilk in medium bowl and mix until smooth. Add dry ingredients and stir with a wire whisk until creamy. Refrigerate to thicken and blend flavors.

Yield: 2 cups

Oil and Lemon Dressing

- ¼ c. olive oil
- ¼ c. fresh lemon juice
- ¼ t. salt
- freshly ground black pepper
- 2 T. fresh parsley, minced

Combine all ingredients in a small bowl or cruet. Shake or stir well before serving.

Yield: ½ cup

Honey-Mustard Dressing

- 1 T. Dijon-style mustard
- 3 T. honey
- 3 T. fresh lemon juice
- ½ t. salt
- ½ t. freshly ground black pepper
- ½ c. vegetable oil

Combine mustard, honey, lemon juice, salt and pepper in medium bowl. Whisk together until smooth. Gradually whisk in oil to form a creamy dressing.

Yield: 1 cup

Poppy Seed Dressing for Fruit

- ¼ c. vegetable oil
- ¼ c. lime juice
- 2 T. sugar
- dash red pepper sauce (Tabasco)
- 2 t. poppy seeds

Combine all ingredients in tightly covered jar or cruet. Shake well to blend. Serve over prepared fresh fruit.

Yield: ½ cup

Ranch Dressing

- ½ c. regular or light mayonnaise
- ½ c. buttermilk
- ¼ t. each onion powder, garlic powder, black pepper
- ½ t. salt
- ½ t. sugar
- 1 t. dry parsley, crushed

Combine mayonnaise and buttermilk. Add seasonings and stir to combine. Refrigerate to thicken and blend flavors.

Yield: 1 cup

Reduced Fat Ranch Dressing

- ¼ c. regular or light mayonnaise
- ¾ c. buttermilk
- ¼ t. each onion powder, garlic powder, black pepper
- ½ t. salt
- ½ t. sugar
- 1 t. dry parsley, crushed
- 2-3 t. E-Z Gel®

Combine mayonnaise and buttermilk. Add seasonings and stir to combine. Gradually add E-Z Gel®, stirring constantly with wire whisk. Refrigerate to thicken and blend flavors.

Yield: 1 cup

Dill Dressing

- ½ c. light mayonnaise
- 1½ c. buttermilk
- ½ t. onion powder
- ½ t. garlic powder
- 1 t. salt
- 1 t. sugar
- 1½ T. E-Z Gel®

- 2 t. dried dill weed (NOT dill seed)
- 1 t. dried parsley, crushed, OR 2 t. fresh parsley, washed and snipped

Combine mayonnaise and buttermilk in medium bowl and mix until smooth. Add dry ingredients and stir with a wire whisk until creamy. Refrigerate to thicken and blend flavors.

Yield: 2 cups

Soups, Stews, and Savory Sauces

Soups

Beef Stock

- 1 T. vegetable oil
- 3 lbs. meaty beef bones
- 1 medium onion, trimmed and quartered
- 1 carrot, peeled and chopped
- 1 stalk celery with leaves, chopped
- 1 garlic cloves
- 1-2 c. water
- 1 bay leaves
- ½ t. salt
- ¼ t. ground pepper

Preheat oven to 450°. Pour oil into a large roasting pan and heat briefly in the oven. Add the bones to the oil in the pan, turning to coat lightly with oil, and roast for 30 minutes. Add the onion, carrot and celery, tossing lightly to coat with oil. Roast 30 minutes longer. Remove the pan from the oven and transfer the bones and vegetables to a large stockpot. Drain off as much fat as possible.

Place the roasting pan over medium-high heat and add water. Boil briefly to release browned bits of meat and vegetables. Add this liquid to the bones and vegetables in the stock pot with enough cold water to cover. Bring to a boil, skimming residual foam that forms. Reduce heat and add seasonings. Simmer uncovered for 6-8 hours, adding water as necessary.

Strain stock through a colander lined with a double layer of cheesecloth or heavy paper towel.

Stock may be used immediately or stored for later use. If you wish to remove more of the fat from the broth, refrigerate over night and remove fat cap. To store, pour stock into airtight containers. Label, date and refrigerate for up to three days or freeze for up to six months.

Uses for beef stock: Base for beef stew or soups. Use in place of water when making rice for a richer flavor. Warm and sip for a sore throat.

Yield: 1-2 quarts

Chicken or Turkey Stock

- 3 lb. chicken or turkey parts (backs, necks, carcasses, giblets except liver, etc.)
- 1 large onion
- 1 carrot, peeled and chopped
- 1 stalk celery with leaves, chopped
- 1 garlic clove, crushed
- 2 T. fresh parsley
- ½ t. dried thyme
- 1 bay leaf
- ½ t. salt
- ¼ t. ground pepper

Wash chicken parts and place in a large stockpot. For a richer flavor brown chicken bits, then add cold water to cover chicken. Bring to a boil, skimming the froth from the surface as it forms. Reduce heat and add chopped vegetables and seasonings. Simmer, uncovered, for three hours, adding water as necessary.

Strain stock through a colander lined with a double layer of cheesecloth or heavy paper towel. Stock may be used immediately or stored for later use. To store, pour stock into airtight containers. Label, date and refrigerate for up to three days or freeze for up to six months.

Yield: 1-2 quarts

Beef Gravy from Drippings

Remove pot roast from pan. Deglaze pan, stirring well to remove crusty bits. Skim to remove excess fat. Add additional water and beef base for desired amount of gravy (allow ¼-½ c. broth per person). Bring broth to a gentle boil. Prepare a slurry of water and starch (2 T. flour plus water to thin OR 1 T. ThickGel® or cornstarch with water to thin for every cup of broth). Gradually add slurry to boiling broth, stirring constantly. Return to a boil and simmer gently for about 5 minutes.

*May also use homemade stock, canned broth, mixture of bouillon and water, or a combination of any of the above.

If a lighter gravy is desired replace beef drippings with drippings from roasted chicken or turkey and follow directions as above.

Gravies can be spiced with salt, pepper, herbs, and liquid smoke depending on your desired flavor profile.

Note: Thickening with flour makes an opaque, country-style gravy. Cornstarch makes a translucent gravy without a "floury" taste. If a heartier cornstarch gravy is desired a small amount of milk or cream may be added just before serving.

Gravy is a great addition to freezer meals as it can be used over rice or potatoes to seal out air and freezer burn.

Hamburger Soup

- 1 lb. lean ground beef
- ½ c. diced onion
- 2 c. baby carrots, cut in halves
- 2 c. diced potatoes
- 2 (15 oz.) can diced tomatoes
- 1 t. salt
- 1/8 t. pepper
- ¼ c. E-Z Gel®

Place ground beef in heavy six-quart stockpot. Turn stove to medium heat and brown beef through, remove excess grease. Add onion, carrots and potatoes and sauté for three minutes. Reduce heat and stir in tomatoes and seasonings. Cover and cook over low heat until vegetables are tender (20-25 minutes). Gradually stir in E-Z Gel® or simmer to reduce. Heat to serving temperature. Serve with bread or Utah scones.

Yield: 8 servings

Beef Stew

- 1 T. olive or canola oil
- 1 lb. lean stew meat, visible fat removed and cut into 1" cubes
- 2 c. water
- ½ t. each garlic powder and onion powder
- 2 t. low sodium beef base or bouillon cubes

- ½ - 1 t. salt
- ¼ t. ground black pepper
- 1 medium onion, chopped
- 2 large potatoes, peeled and cubed
- 2 cups baby carrots, halved
- 2 cups water
- 1 (16 oz.) can green beans, drained
- 6-8 T. E-Z Gel®
- 5 oz. frozen peas

Heat olive oil in heavy 6-quart Dutch oven over medium high heat. Add stew meat and cook, stirring frequently, until meat is well browned on all sides. Add water, garlic powder, onion powder, beef base, salt, pepper and 2 cups water. Cover tightly and simmer, adding water if needed, for 1½ hours or until meat is tender. Add onion, potatoes, carrots and an additional 2 c. water. Cover and simmer for an additional 30 minutes until vegetables are tender. Push meat and vegetables to the side of the pan and gradually add E-Z Gel®, stirring with a wire whisk until gravy is smooth. Alternatively, simmer to reduce or add a cornstarch slurry made from 1 T. cornstarch and 2-3 T. water. Season to taste. Stir in green beans and frozen peas. Simmer 5 minutes more.

Serve immediately or divide into freezer containers. Seal, label, date and freeze for up to three months. This recipe also makes a great filling for pot pie.

Yield: 8 servings

Easy Cream of Broccoli Soup

- 1 c. water
- 2 t. chicken base
- ¼ c. chopped onion
- 1 c. chopped broccoli (fresh or frozen)
- 2 c. milk
- 4 T. flour OR 2 T. cornstarch OR 2 T. ThickGel®
- ½ c. grated cheddar cheese (opt.)

Combine water and chicken base in a medium saucepan. Add onion and broccoli, cover, and cook over medium heat until vegetables are tender (about 5 minutes). Combine milk with starch in a quart jar and shake until mixture is smooth. Gradually add to simmering broccoli mixture, stirring constantly with wire whisk. Cook until smooth and creamy. Remove from heat and add grated cheese and stir until cheese is melted. Season to taste with salt and pepper.

Yield: 4 cups

Note: Other vegetables (or a combination of several) may be substituted for, or added to, the broccoli i.e., mushrooms, cauliflower, potatoes, carrots, etc.

Traditional Cream of Broccoli Soup

- 1 c. chopped broccoli (fresh or frozen)
- 1 c. water
- 1 t. chicken base
- 3 T. butter or margarine
- ¼ c. chopped onion
- 3 T. flour
- 2 c. milk

Combine water, and chicken base in a medium saucepan. Add broccoli, cover, and cook over medium heat until tender (about 5 minutes). Meanwhile melt butter or margarine in frying pan. Add onions and cook over medium heat until onions are limp and clear. Add flour and stir well. Cook over low heat for about three minutes until roux is well formed and light tan. Stir to prevent scorching. Remove from heat and add milk all at once, stirring constantly. Return to heat and cook until thick, stirring well. Add milk mixture to cooked broccoli-broth mixture and heat through. Serve immediately.

Yield: 4 cups

Note: Other vegetables (or a combination of several) may be substituted for the broccoli i.e. mushrooms, cauliflower, potatoes, carrots, etc.

Chicken Stew

- 1 lb. chicken pieces with bones
- 4 c. water
- 1 t. chicken base or 1 bouillon cube
- ½ medium onion, quartered
- tops of 2 stalks celery
- 1 bay leaf
- 2 carrots, peeled and sliced
- 3 medium potatoes, peeled and diced
- ¼ c. flour
- ½ c. water
- ½ c. frozen peas

Combine chicken, water, chicken base, onion, celery, and bay leaf in 6-quart Dutch oven. Bring to a boil over high heat, then cover and reduce heat to low. Simmer gently for 30-45 minutes until chicken is fork-tender. Remove chicken and set aside. Strain broth, removing vegetables and bay leaf. Return broth to Dutch oven and add prepared carrots and potatoes. Cook until tender–about 8 minutes. Meanwhile, remove cooked chicken pieces from bones and cut into bite-sized chunks. Combine flour and water in a small bowl to form a slurry. Stir well to remove all lumps. Gradually add slurry to cooking vegetable mixture, stirring constantly until thick. Gently fold in chicken pieces and frozen peas. Heat through.

Yield: 6-8 servings

Chicken Noodle Soup

- 1 lb. chicken pieces with bones
- 4 c. water
- 1 t. chicken base or 1 bouillon cube
- ½ medium onion, quartered
- tops of 2 stalks celery
- 1 bay leaf
- 2 carrots, peeled and sliced
- 3 medium potatoes, peeled and diced
- ½ c. frozen peas
- Egg Noodles, see Grains, Pasta, and Legumes section

Combine chicken, water, chicken base, onion, celery, and bay leaf in 6-quart Dutch oven. Bring to a boil over high heat, then cover and reduce heat to low. Simmer gently for 30-45 minutes until chicken is fork-tender. Remove chicken and set aside. Strain broth, removing vegetables and bay leaf. Return broth to Dutch oven and add prepared carrots and potatoes. Cook until tender–about 8 minutes. Meanwhile, remove cooked chicken pieces from bones and cut into bite-sized chunks. Gently fold in chicken pieces, cooked noodles, and frozen peas. Heat through.

Yield: 6-8 servings

Clam Chowder

- 2 potatoes, peeled and cubed
- 1 stalk celery, trimmed and diced
- ½ medium onion, peeled and diced
- 2 c. chicken broth
- 4 T. butter or margarine
- 4 T. flour
- 1 c. cream
- 1 c. milk
- 1 can minced or chopped clams

Combine potatoes, celery, onion, chicken broth, and the juice from the clams in a medium saucepan. Bring to a boil. Reduce heat and simmer for 15-20 minutes until vegetables are tender. Melt butter in medium frying pan. Add flour. Cook, stirring constantly, 1 minute. Whisk in cream and milk and heat until thickened. Add thickened milk mixture and clams to vegetables. Return to serving temperature over low heat, stirring to prevent scorching. Season to taste with salt and pepper.

This can be topped with bacon bits, chives, and a little bit of cheese for additional flavor and color.

Yield: 4 servings

Sauces

Alfredo Sauce

- ¼ c. butter
- 2 c. cream
- ½ t. salt
- ¼ t. ground pepper
- ¾ c. freshly grated Parmesan cheese

Combine butter, cream, salt and pepper in skillet. Bring to a gentle boil; reduce heat and simmer 4 minutes, stirring to prevent scorching. Stir in Parmesan cheese and heat through. Do not boil. Mixture will be thin. Serve with cooked fettuccine noodles.

Yield: 4 servings

Lower-fat Alfredo

Melt 1 T. butter in medium saucepan. Add 1 T. flour. Cook, stirring constantly, 1 minute. Whisk in 1 c. milk, 1 c. cream, ¾ t. salt and ¼ t. ground pepper. Bring to a gentle boil, stirring constantly. Reduce heat and simmer, stirring occasionally, 4 minutes. Stir in ¾ c. freshly grated Parmesan cheese and heat through. Do not boil Serve with cooked drained fettuccine noodles.

Yield: 4 servings

White Sauce (layman's White Country Gravy)

- 2 T. butter
- 2 T. all-purpose flour
- 2 c. milk
- 3 T. E-Z Gel®
- salt and pepper

Melt butter in a heavy saucepan over medium heat. Add flour all at once and stir until combined. Continue to cook, stirring constantly until bubbly and light tan. Add milk gradually, stirring with a wire whisk. Gradually add E-Z Gel®, stirring with a wire whisk. Season to taste and continue cooking until sauce thickens.

Replace E-Z Gel® by doubling the butter and the flour.

Yield: 2 cups

Cheese Sauce

- 2 cups White Sauce
- ½ c. shredded cheese
- salt and pepper to taste

Heat prepared white sauce. Stir in cheese until melted. Season to taste with salt and pepper, herbs or spices. Serve over vegetables, or combine with pasta for quick mac and cheese. It may be necessary to thin the sauce with a little milk to reach the desired consistency.

Yield: 2 ½ cups sauce

Mornay Sauce

- 2 c. milk
- 2 T. minced onion
- 1 small bay leaf.
- 4 T. butter
- 4 T. flour
- 2 T. heavy cream
- ¼ c. Parmesan cheese
- ¼ c. grated Swiss cheese

Combine milk, onion and bay leaf in a medium saucepan. Bring to a gentle boil, but do not scorch. Remove from heat and let stand 10 minutes. Strain. Melt butter in saucepan. Add flour and cook until light brown. Gradually add prepared milk mixture and cream, stirring constantly until mixture starts to boil. Stir in salt and pepper to taste. Cook over low heat, stirring often, about 5 minutes. Sprinkle in cheese. Stir until melted and smooth. Serve with pasta, eggs, vegetables or fish.

Yield: 4 servings

Mushroom Sauce

- ¼ c. butter
- 1 c. fresh mushrooms, washed and sliced
- 2 T. minced onion
- ¼ c. flour
- 1 t. chicken bouillon
- 2 c. milk OR part milk, part cream
- salt and pepper to taste

Melt butter in medium saucepan. Sauté mushrooms and onion until tender, 3-4 minutes. Stir in flour and cook until light brown. Gradually add milk and bring to a gently boil, stirring constantly to prevent lumping and avoid scorching. Season to taste. Serve with pasta, chicken, vegetables, or eggs.

Yield: 4 servings

Curry Sauce for Chicken or Turkey

- ¼ c. butter or margarine
- 1 clove garlic, minced
- 1 onion, chopped
- 1 apple, peeled, cored and chopped
- 1 t. curry powder
- ¼ c. flour or ThickGel®
- 1 c. chicken broth
- ½ c. cream
- ½ c. milk
- salt and pepper to taste

Sauté garlic, onion and apple in butter for about 5 minutes. Stir in the curry powder and flour and cook 1 minute more. Add chicken broth, milk, and cream, stirring constantly, and return to a boil. Season to taste with salt and pepper. Serve with cooked chicken or turkey (the meat can be on the side, or folded into the sauce) over rice.

Yield: 2 cups

Sweet and Sour Sauce

- ½ c. sugar
- ½ c. chicken broth or water
- ¼ c. white vinegar
- 1 t. vegetable oil
- 1 t soy sauce
- ¼ t. salt
- 1 clove crushed garlic
- 2 T. cornstarch
- 2 T. water
- 1 tomato, cut into thin wedges
- 1 small green pepper, cut into 1" pieces
- 1 20-oz. can pineapple chunks, drained

Combine sugar, broth, vinegar, oil, soy sauce, salt, and garlic in small sauce pan. Bring to a gentle boil over medium heat. Thicken with mixture of cornstarch and water, stirring constantly. Add remaining ingredients and return to a boil. Serve hot.

Yield: 2½ cups sauce

Homemade Barbecue Sauce

- 2 T. butter
- 1 medium onion, sliced
- 1 clove garlic, minced
- ¾ c. water
- 1 c. catsup
- 2 T. EACH vinegar and lemon juice
- ¼ c. brown sugar
- 1 t. salt
- ¼ t. pepper
- 2 T. Worcestershire sauce
- 1 T. dry mustard
- 2 t. liquid smoke

Sauté onion and garlic in melted butter. Add other ingredients and cook over medium heat for 20 minutes.

Yield: 2 cups

Pasta and Legumes

Pasta

Tuna-Noodle Casserole

- 1 10¾-oz. can condensed cream of mushroom OR cream of chicken soup
- ½ c. water
- 1 c. grated cheddar cheese
- 1 6-oz. can tuna in water, drained
- 1 c. frozen peas
- 6 ounces noodles, **cooked and drained**
- salt and pepper to taste

Combine soup, water and cheese in a medium saucepan. Heat gently, stirring occasionally until cheese is melted. Fold in tuna, peas and cooked noodles. Heat through. Season to taste. Garnish with crushed potato chips.

Yield: 4 servings

Baked Tuna-Noodle Casserole

2 T. butter

- 1 small onion, chopped
- 2 T. flour
- ½ c. sour cream
- ½ c. milk
- ½ c. grated cheese
- 1 6-oz. can tuna, drained
- ½ t. salt
- 6 ounces noodles, **cooked and drained**
- ½ c. crushed cornflakes
- 1 T. melted butter or margarine

Preheat oven to 350°. Butter a 2 quart casserole dish. Melt the butter in a skillet and cook the onion over medium heat. Add flour, stirring constantly, and cook until mixture is a light brown. Add sour cream and milk and heat until thickened. Stir in cheese, tuna and salt. Gently fold noodles into sauce until mixed. Turn into prepared casserole dish. Combine cornflakes and melted butter and sprinkle over the top of the casserole. Bake for 30 minutes.

Yield: 4 servings

Homemade Macaroni and Cheese

- 2 T. margarine or butter
- 2 T. flour
- 1½ c. milk
- 1 c. grated cheddar cheese
- salt and pepper to taste
- 6-8 ounces macaroni, cooked and drained
- ¼ c. bread crumbs (opt.)
- 1 t. melted butter (opt.)

Melt butter in medium frying pan. Add flour and stir constantly until mixture bubbles and turns a light tan color. Add milk and heat to a boil over medium heat, stirring constantly until thickened. Reduce heat to low and fold in cheese to form a creamy cheese sauce. Method 1: Fold cooked pasta into sauce. Serve immediately. Method 2: Put cooked macaroni in 1½ quart casserole dish and pour the cheese sauce over. Mix gently to combine. Sprinkle with mixture of bread crumbs and melted butter. Bake uncovered at 375° F. for 30 minutes until bubbly.

Yield: 4 servings

Hot Buttered Spaghetti

- 8 ounces spaghetti
- 1 T. butter
- 1 T. olive oil
- 2 cloves minced garlic

- ¼ c. chopped fresh parsley
- salt and pepper to taste
- ½ c. freshly grated Parmesan cheese

Cook spaghetti in 4 quarts boiling salted water just until tender, about 8 minutes. Meanwhile heat butter, olive oil and garlic in a small saucepan until mixture is hot. Remove from heat and stir in parsley. Drain spaghetti and return immediately to pan. Toss with butter mixture and Parmesan cheese; season as desired. Serve hot.

Yield: 4 servings.

Homemade Egg Noodles

- 1 c. flour (can substitute part semolina flour)
- ¼ t. salt and a dash pepper
- 2 eggs, well beaten
- 1-2 t. water

Pour flour into a pile on a wooden cutting board. With hands, stir in salt and pepper. Form a well in the center of the flour pile and add eggs. Manipulate with hands until egg is fully incorporated into the flour mixture. Add a little water, a few drops at a time, to form a stiff, smooth dough. Knead well. Cover with plastic wrap and let stand 5 minutes. Roll very thin and cut into strips about ¼" thick. Cook immediately in 6 quarts boiling salted water or let dry on wooden pasta rack until firm and refrigerate for up to three days.

Yield: 4 servings

Pasta Salad with Vegetables

- 8 ounces rigatoni noodles
- 1 tomato, diced
- 4 radishes, sliced
- ½ c. broccoli, chopped
- 1 carrot, thinly sliced
- 1 green onion, thinly sliced
- ¼ c. sliced ripe olives
- Italian dressing to taste.

Cook noodles in 5 quarts rapidly boiling salted water just until tender, about 9 minutes. Drain and rinse under cold water to chill. Pour cooled pasta into a medium bowl and toss with remaining ingredients. Refrigerate for 30 minutes to allow flavors to absorb. Toss again before serving.

Yield: 4 servings

Legumes

Brad's Baked Beans

- ¼ pound ground beef
- 2 slices bacon, cubed
- 1 T. chopped onion
- 1 T. chopped green pepper
- 1 15½-oz. can pork and beans
- 1 15½-oz can other beans (garbanzo, black, kidney, pinto, chili, etc.), drained
- 2 slices pineapple, cut into chunks (opt.)
- 3 T. molasses
- 3 T. brown sugar
- ½ c. barbecue sauce

Brown ground beef and bacon in frying pan. Remove meats and reserve. Drain all but 1 T. fat. Add onion and green pepper to pan and sauté until onion is tender. Method 1: Combine all ingredients in a medium casserole dish; cover and bake for 1 hour. Method 2: Combine all ingredients in heavy Dutch oven. Cover and simmer on low heat, stirring occasionally, for 30 minutes.

Yield: 4 servings

Chili with Beans

- ½ lb. ground beef
- ½ medium onion, chopped
- 1 small clove garlic, minced
- ½ t. salt
- ½ t. paprika
- 1 T. chili powder (mild)
- 1 t. cumin
- red pepper flakes to taste (opt.)
- 2 t. cornstarch or ThickGel®
- 1 14½-oz. cans stewed tomatoes
- 1 15½ -oz. cans kidney or small red beans, drained and rinsed

Brown ground beef in Dutch oven with onion and garlic. Drain excess grease. Combine salt, spices, cornstarch, and stewed tomatoes. Add tomato mixture and beans and simmer for 1 hour. Adjust seasonings to taste. Serve hot.

Yield: 4 servings

Taco Soup

- ½ lb. lean ground beef
- ½ medium onion, chopped
- 1 clove garlic, minced
- 1 T. chili powder (mild)
- ½ t. salt
- ½ t. paprika
- 1 t. cumin
- ¼-½ t. red pepper flakes
- 2 t. cornstarch or ThickGel®
- 2 14½-oz. cans stewed tomatoes
- 1 15½-oz. can kidney or small red beans, drained and rinsed
- 1 c. frozen corn (canned works as well, but not creamed)

Brown ground beef in large saucepan with onion and garlic. Drain excess grease. Combine salt, spices, cornstarch, and stewed tomatoes. Add tomato mixture and beans to meat mixture and simmer for ten to fifteen minutes. Add frozen corn and heat to serving temperature. Adjust seasonings. Serve with tortilla chips and garnish with cheese, sour cream, olives, and green onion.

Yield: 4-6 servings

Goulash

- ¼ pound ground beef
- 2 T. chopped onion
- ½ t. garlic powder
- 1 t. Italian seasoning
- 1 14½-oz. can stewed tomatoes
- 1 8-oz. can tomato sauce
- 1 15½-oz. can small red beans
- 4 ounces cooked pasta
- ½ c. grated cheddar cheese
- salt and pepper to taste

Brown ground beef and onion in Dutch oven. Season with garlic powder and Italian seasoning. Stir in tomatoes, tomato sauce, and red beans and simmer over low heat for 20 minutes, stirring occasionally. Fold in cooked pasta and cheese and heat until the cheese is melted.

Yield: 4-6 servings

Main Dishes: Beef and Pork

Beef

Ground Beef Stroganoff

- ½ pound ground beef
- 2 T. chopped onion
- 1 T. dried onion soup mix
- 1 10 ¾-oz. can condensed cream of mushroom soup
- 1 cup water
- 1 4-oz. can sliced mushrooms (opt.)
- ¼ cup sour cream
- 6-8 ounces noodles, cooked and drained

Brown ground beef in skillet; drain excess grease. Add onion and cook until onion is soft. Add soups, water and mushrooms and stir well. Simmer on low heat for 10-15 minutes. Add sour cream just before serving. Do not boil. Serve over hot cooked noodles.

Yield : 4 servings

Spaghetti with Meat Sauce

- ½ pound ground beef
- 2 T. onion, chopped
- 1 clove garlic, minced
- 1 8-oz. can tomato sauce
- 1 14½-oz. can diced or stewed tomatoes
- 1 t. sugar
- ½ t. crushed oregano
- ½ t. Italian Seasoning
- salt and pepper to taste
- 6-8 ounces spaghetti noodles, cooked and drained

Brown ground beef in skillet. Drain excess grease. Add onion and garlic and cook until onion is soft. Stir in tomato sauce and tomatoes. Add seasonings and simmer on low heat for 15-20 minutes. Adjust seasonings. If desired, sauce may be thickened with a mixture of 2 t. cornstarch and 2 T. water or a small amount of E-Z Gel®. Serve over hot cooked noodles.

This sauce works great in lasagna as well.

Yield: 4 servings

Tacos

Brown 1 lb. lean ground beef in heavy frying pan over medium heat. Reduce heat to low and stir in one batch of taco seasoning mix (recipe below) and 1/4-1/2 cup water. Simmer gently. Add up to 15 ounce of drained black beans if desired. Serve with tortillas or taco shells, cheese, lettuce, tomatoes, salsa, the works!

Yield: 8 servings

Taco Seasoning Mix

- 2 t. mild chili powder
- ½ t. paprika
- ½ t. salt
- 1 t. ground cumin
- ½ t. ground black pepper
- 1 t. onion powder
- ½ t. garlic powder
- ¼-½ t. red pepper flakes (opt.)
- 1 T. E-Z Gel®

Measure ingredients into a small plastic snack-sized bag. Shake well to combine. Seal, label, and date or use immediate in tacos or fajitas.

Yield: one packet

Sweet and Sour Meatballs

Meatballs:

- 1 lb. ground beef
- 2 T. E-Z Gel® modified food starch OR ¼ c. dried bread crumbs
- 2 T. dried minced onion
- ½ t. salt and ¼ t. pepper

Sauce:

- 1 (20 oz.) can pineapple chunks
- ¼ c. sugar
- 2 T. soy sauce
- 2 T. vinegar
- ½ c. water
- 4 T. E-Z Gel® modified food starch
- 1-2 green peppers, sliced

Preheat oven to 400° F. Combine meatball ingredients in small bowl. Do not overmix!!! Shape into 1" balls and place in baking pan. Bake 12 minutes. Drain well.

Combine juice from pineapple chunks, sugar, soy sauce, vinegar, and water in medium bowl. Gradually add E-Z Gel®, stirring constantly with wire whisk. Add pineapple and stir to combine. Pour over meatballs in baking pan, then lay sliced peppers on top. Bake for 20 minutes at 375° until peppers are crisp-tender. Serve over rice.

Yield: 4 servings

Porcupine Meatballs

- 1 lb. ground beef
- 1 egg, slightly beaten
- ½ c. uncooked rice
- 1 t. salt
- ½ t. pepper
- 1 T. minced dried onion
- 1 can (10½ oz.) condensed tomato soup
- 1 can (10½ oz.) water

Combine first six ingredients and shape into meatballs. Method 1: Heat soup and water in pressure saucepan to a gentle boil. Add meatballs, then lid the pressure saucepan and cook at 15 lbs. pressure for 10 minutes. Remove from heat and cool for 5 minutes then run under tap water to reduce pressure. Remove pressure gauge, then lid. Serve. Method 2: Combine soup and 1¼ c. water in medium casserole dish. Add meatballs, then cover and bake 45 minutes. Method 3: Heat soup and water in medium saucepan. Add meatballs. Cover with tight lid and cook on medium low heat for about 30 minutes, stirring occasionally.

Yield: 4 servings

Swiss Steak

- 1 lb. round steak cut into four pieces
- ½ c. flour
- ¼ t. salt
- dash pepper
- ½ t. herb chicken seasoning
- 2 T. vegetable oil
- 1 medium onion, sliced
- 2 c. water
- 2 t. beef base OR 2 beef bouillon cubes

Combine flour and seasonings in flat pan. Dredge steak pieces in seasoned flour mixture and pound with meat mallet until steaks are about _" thick and flour is pounded into the meat.

Heat 2 T. oil in heavy frying pan. Add meat, one or two pieces at a time to avoid crowding, and brown well on both sides. Method 1: Remove browned meat to pressure saucepan. Layer with sliced onions. Add water and beef base to frying pan and return to heat, stirring to remove crusty bits. Pour broth mixture over browned meat and seal with lid. Bring to 15 lbs. pressure over high heat, then reduce heat until the weight rocks gently and hisses 3-5 times per minute. Cook for 15-20 minutes. Remove from heat and cool. Remove pressure gauge, then lid. Season broth as necessary, then thicken broth with flour slurry. Method 2: Place browned meat in medium casserole dish. Layer with sliced onions. Add 3 c. water and beef base to frying pan and return to heat, stirring to remove crusty bits. Pour broth mixture over browned meat. Bake in oven, covered, for 1-2 hours. Method 3: Layer with sliced onion and cover with mixture of water and beef base. Cover with tight lid and cook for about 1-2 hours, adding additional liquid as needed.

Yield: 4 servings

Marinated Beef

- 1 t. finely grated fresh ginger
- 1 t. minced garlic
- 1 t. chopped green onion
- 1 t. sesame oil
- 1-2 t. toasted sesame seeds
- 3 T. soy sauce
- 1½ t. sugar
- ¼ t. ground black pepper
- 1 lb. thinly sliced beef

Combine ingredients in a medium bowl and marinate overnight or at least 1 hour. Stir fry in a large frying pan or wok over medium high heat. Serve with hot cooked rice.

Yield: 4 servings

Steak 'n Stuff Pitas

- 1 large ripe tomato
- 1 lb. boneless sirloin steak, thinly sliced
- 1 T. vegetable oil
- 8 oz. mushrooms, sliced
- 1 large onion, thinly sliced
- ½ each green and red bell peppers, sliced
- 1½ t. Italian seasoning
- ½ t. garlic powder
- Salt and pepper to taste
- 1 c. shredded mozzarella cheese
- 2 T. dairy sour cream
- 4 homemade (or purchased) pitas, halved
- Curly endive (opt.)
- Bell pepper rings (opt.)

Remove tomato peel from tomato in one long continuous strip. Shape into rose and reserve for garnish. Dice tomato; reserve.

Heat oil in heavy frying pan over medium-high heat. Add half of the sliced beef and stir fry 4-6 minutes until brown. Remove from pan with slotted spoon, set aside, and repeat with remaining meat. Stir fry mushrooms and onion in pan drippings over medium high heat for 2-3 minutes, adding a few drops of water if necessary to prevent sticking. Add green and red bell pepper and stir fry until onions are transparent, peppers are crisp-tender, and moisture is absorbed.

Return beef to pan. Sprinkle with Italian seasoning, garlic powder, and salt and pepper to taste and mix well. Stir in cheese and sour cream; reduce heat to low. Cover and cook 1-2 minutes until cheese melts. Stir in reserved chopped tomato and cook 1 more minute. Fill pita bread halves (page 238) with beef mixture and arrange on platter lined with curly endive. Garnish platter with tomato rose and bell pepper slices.

Yield: 4 servings

Jack-o-lantern Burgers

- 1 lb, ground beef
- 2 T. E-Z Gel®
- 1 T, dried chopped onion
- 1/2 t. salt and a dash of pepper
- 1/4 c. chunky salsa
- Cheese slices

Combine all ingredients except cheese slices, mixing lightly. Do not overmix. An egg can be added for increased moisture. Shape into hamburger patties and grill or fry until well browned on both sides and cooked through. Cut pumpkin faces into cheese slices and place on browned hamburgers, cooking an additional 2-3 minutes or until cheese melts.

Yield: 4 servings

Roast Beef

- 2 lb. beef chuck roast
- 2 T. flour
- 1 t. salt
- dash pepper
- 1 T. vegetable oil
- 1 pkg. onion soup mix
- 2 c. water

Combine flour and seasonings and coat roast with mixture. Heat oil in heavy frying pan or pressure saucepan and brown meat on all sides over medium high heat. Method 1: Place meat, soup mix and water in 6-quart pressure saucepan and cook at 15 lbs. pressure for 45 minutes. Remove from heat and cool for 5 minutes, then run under cool tap water to reduce pressure. Adjust seasonings as necessary and thicken broth with flour or cornstarch slurry. To add vegetables, pressure meat for 30 minutes, then run under cool tap water to reduce pressure. Add potatoes and carrots to pressure saucepan and return to pressure for 5 minutes. Run under tap water to reduce pressure. Remove meat and vegetables to platter and thicken broth for gravy. Method 2: Place meat, soup mix, and 3 cups water in an oven-safe baking pan. Cover tightly and bake at 350°, for 3 hours. Add vegetables for last hour, if desired. Method 3: Place meat, soup mix, and water in heavy Dutch oven. Cover with tight fitting lid and cook for 2-3 hours, adding liquid as needed. Add vegetables for last 30 minutes if desired.

Yield: 6 servings

Egg Rolls

- ½ lb. lean ground beef
- ½ t. finely grated gingerroot
- 1 clove garlic, minced
- 1 c. finely chopped cabbage
- ½ c. shredded carrot
- ¼ c. finely chopped onion
- 2 T. soy sauce
- ½ t. sugar
- ¼ t. salt
- 10 egg roll wrappers

Fry ground beef, gingerroot, and garlic over medium high heat until meat is no longer pink. Add vegetables and cook mixture until tender. Season to taste with soy sauce, sugar and salt. Cool. Lay egg roll wrapper on flat surface at a diagonal. Place a large spoonful of filling just below the center. Fold top corner over filling, tucking under on the opposite side. Fold side corners over filling, forming an envelop shape. Brush edges of wrapper lightly with water, then finish rolling to seal. Repeat with remaining wrappers and filling.

Heat least 2 inches vegetable oil in a heavy saucepan, wok, or deep-fat fryer to 375° F. Fry egg rolls, a few at a time, until golden brown. Drain on paper towels. Keep warm in 300° F oven until serving. Serve with sweet-and-sour sauce.

Yield: 10 egg rolls

Spring Rolls

- 1 lb. ground beef
- 1 T. vegetable oil
- ¾ lb. bean sprouts
- 1 head green cabbage, chopped
- 1 bunch green onions, sliced
- 2 carrots, grated
- 3 T. soy sauce
- 2 t. black pepper
- 1 c. water
- 1 egg, slightly beaten
- 20 egg rolls wrappers
- vegetable oil

Brown ground beef in heavy frying pan over medium high heat. Drain fat and set meat aside. Add vegetable oil to frying pan and stir fry vegetables until limp, then add the browned beef, soy sauce, pepper, and water and cook until vegetables are done and moisture is absorbed. Let cool for 10 minutes. Wrap in egg roll wrappers as directed on package, brushing edges lightly with water to seal. Deep fry over medium heat. Drain and serve with Sweet and Sour Sauce (Soups, Stews, and Savory Sauces Chapter).

Yield: 20 spring rolls

Pork

Pan-fried Pork Chops

- 4 pork chops
- salt and pepper to taste
- chicken herb seasoning as desired
- ¼ c. water

Heat large frying pan to approximate 375°. Add chops and brown on both sides, seasoning as desired. Add water and cover with tight-fitting lid, then reduce heat and simmer for 10 minutes, adding additional water if needed to prevent scorching.

Yield: 4 servings

Barbecued Ribs

- 2 lbs. country style boneless pork spareribs
- 3 cups water
- 1 bay leaf
- ½ onion, quartered
- 1 (18-oz) bottle prepared barbecue sauce OR 2 c. homemade barbecue sauce (Soups, Stews, and Savory Sauce Chapter)
- ¼ c. brown sugar
- 1 medium onion, sliced
- 4 oz. mushrooms, sliced
- 1 medium green pepper, sliced

Trim excess fat from spareribs, then place in 6-quart Dutch oven with water, bay leaf, and onion. Simmer over medium heat for 40 minutes (20 minutes at 15 lbs. in pressure saucepan). Remove ribs and discard broth. Place ribs in medium saucepan with barbecue sauce and brown sugar. Cover and simmer over medium heat for 30 minutes or more until tender. Add sliced onion and mushrooms and cook for 5 minutes more. Stir in green pepper slices and cook just until crisp-tender. Serve with hot cooked rice.

Yield: 4 servings

Main Dishes: Chicken and Seafood

Chicken

Fajita or Taco Seasoning Mix

- 1 T. chili powder (mild)
- ½ t. salt and a dash of black pepper
- 1 T. dehydrated minced onion
- ½ t. paprika
- 1 t. cumin
- 2 t. cornstarch or E-Z Gel®
- ¼-½ t. red pepper (opt.)

Combine ingredients in small plastic bag. Seal, label, date and store in tightly covered container. For best results use within three months.

Yield: One packet

Chicken Fajitas

- ½ c. water
- ½ c. lime juice
- 1 pkg. fajita or taco seasoning mix (recipe above)
- 2 T. sugar
- 1 lb. boneless skinless chicken breasts
- 2 medium green bell peppers, sliced
- 1 medium red onion, halved and sliced
- 2 T. vegetable oil

Combine first four ingredients in medium bowl. Cut chicken breasts into 1" cubes and marinate in lime juice mixture for at least 15 minutes.

Heat vegetable oil in heavy frying pan over medium high heat. Drain excess marinate from chicken; add chicken to hot pan, stir frying until no longer pink. Add sliced vegetables and stir fry until vegetables are crisp-tender.

Serve on warmed flour tortilla shells with refried beans, chopped tomatoes, grated cheese, sliced olives, diced avocados or prepared guacamole, and sour cream.

Yield: 4-6 servings

Chicken Cordon Bleu

- 4 boneless skinless chicken breasts
- 4 (1-ounce) slices Swiss cheese
- 4 (1-ounce) slices deli ham
- ¼ c. melted butter
- ½ c. dried bread crumbs
- 1 t. chicken herb seasoning
- 2 T. EACH butter and flour
- 1 c. milk
- salt and pepper to taste

Preheat oven to 350°. Place one chicken breast, smooth side down, between two sheets waxed paper or in 1-gallon zippered plastic bag (press air out). Pound with flat end of meat mallet or heavy flat pan to an even thickness–about 3/8". Repeat with remaining chicken pieces. Layer one slice ham and one slice cheese on each chicken breast, then roll up, sealing ham and cheese into the chicken breast. Combine bread crumbs and herb seasoning in a flat container. Dip chicken rolls in melted butter, then into crumb mixture. Arrange in a medium casserole dish and bake for 30-40 minutes until done.

Prepare sauce by making a roux of butter and flour, then adding milk. Return to a boil, stirring constantly until thickened. Season to taste. Serve over hot chicken rolls.

Yield: 4 servings

Chicken A L'Orange

- 4 chicken breast halves
- 1 beaten egg
- 1 T. water
- ¼ c. cornstarch
- 2 T. margarine
- ½ c. brown sugar
- ¼ c. soy sauce
- ½ c. orange juice
- ¼ c. vinegar
- 1 T. cornstarch or ThickGel® in 2 T. water

Dip chicken pieces in egg wash made of beaten egg and water, then coat with cornstarch. Brown in margarine until golden brown and place in shallow baking pan or casserole. Combine remaining ingredients except cornstarch and bring to a boil. Add cornstarch slurry as needed for a thin sauce. Adjust seasonings. Pour over chicken pieces and bake, covered, for 20 minutes, then remove cover and bake an additional 15 minutes.

Yield: 4 servings

Chicken with Orange Glaze

- ½ c. orange juice
- ¼ c. rice wine vinegar
- ½ c. brown sugar
- ¼ c. soy sauce
- ½ t. salt
- 1 t. cornstarch or ThickGel®
- 1 broiler chicken, quartered

Combine first 6 ingredients in medium saucepan and simmer 1 minute. Place chicken quarters in shallow baking pan. Bake at 350° F for 45 minutes, brushing with glaze and turning every 15 minutes.

Serve over hot rice.

Yield: 4 servings

Chicken Mozzarelle

- 2 T. butter
- 2 cloves garlic, pressed or minced
- ½ medium red onion
- ½ lb. fresh mushrooms, sliced
- 4 boneless, skinless chicken or turkey breasts
- ½ t. salt and a dash of pepper
- ½ t. EACH basil and tarragon
- 1 t. Herb Chicken Seasoning
- ¼ c. white grape juice
- ¾ c. chicken broth
- 1 c. grated mozzarella cheese

Melt butter in frying pan. Sauté garlic, onion and mushrooms about 5 minutes, then remove to warm plate. Brown chicken in same frying pan, adding additional butter if needed, until golden brown. Season with salt, pepper, and herbs. Place chicken in casserole dish without overlapping. Pile reserved vegetables over fillets. Add basil, tarragon, grape juice and chicken broth to juices in frying pan and cook for 1 minute, stirring to remove crusty bits. Pour over fillets and vegetables. Cover and bake at 350° F for 30 minutes. Remove cover and sprinkle with shredded cheese. Bake an additional 10 minutes until cheese bubbles. Serve with rice pilaf and steamed vegetables.

Yield: 4 servings

Easy Chicken Enchiladas

- ½ lb. boneless, skinless chicken breast
- 1 10½-oz. can condensed cream of mushroom OR cream or chicken soup
- 2 T. canned diced green chiles
- 1 c. sour cream
- 12 fajita style flour tortillas (purchased or homemade)
- 2 c. grated cheddar cheese

Combine chicken with 2 cups water, ½ t. salt, and 1 T. minced dried onion in medium saucepan. Cook over high heat to a boil, then reduce heat to medium low. Cook for about 10 minutes until chicken is tender and juices run clear. Remove chicken from stock and cool for 5 minutes. Cut into small pieces

Combine soup, chiles, and sour cream. Add ½ c. of soup mixture to chicken. Fill tortillas with chicken mixture and lay in an 8" x 8" casserole dish. Add cheese to remaining soup mixture and

pour over the top. Microwave on high for 10 minutes, then bake at 350° for 10-15 minutes.

Yield: 4 servings

Country Fried Chicken

- 2½ - 3 lb. chicken, cut into pieces
- ½ c. milk or cream
- ¾ c. flour
- 1 t. salt and ½ t. ground pepper
- ½ t. herb chicken seasoning
- ¼ c. butter or margarine
- 1 T. vegetable oil

Wash and dry chicken pieces. Combine flour and seasoning in flat pan. Dip chicken pieces in milk or cream, then dredge well with seasoned flour. Combine butter and oil in large frying pan over medium high heat. When hot, add chicken pieces (dark meat first, then breast pieces a few minutes later) and brown until golden. Reduce heat to medium low, add 1 T. water, cover and cook for about twenty minutes until chicken is no longer pink in the center, checking occasionally to prevent scorching. Remove cover and cook 10 minutes more to crisp. Remove chicken to warm platter and prepare Country Style Chicken Gravy.

Yield: 4 servings

Country Style Chicken Gravy

Add 2 T. butter or margarine to drippings in pan over medium heat, scraping to remove crusty bits. Add 2 T. flour and blend well, then add 1 c. milk or cream. Return to a gentle boil to thicken. Season with salt and pepper and simmer an additional 2 minutes. Adjust seasoning and thickness as desired. Serve with Country Fried Chicken and mashed potatoes.

Yield 4 servings

Chicken and Rice Casserole

- 12 oz. ground sausage
- 1 green pepper, diced
- 1 onion, chopped
- 1 c. chopped celery
- 1 ½ c. rice
- 1 pkg. Lipton Chicken Noodle Soup Mix
- 6 c. hot water
- 2 c. cooked, diced chicken
- ½ c. slivered almonds

Brown sausage in Dutch oven. Add green pepper, onion and celery and sauté 1 minute. Add rice, soup mix, hot water and chicken. Boil for 1 minute. Cover with lid and simmer for 20 minutes. Turn into 9" x 13" baking dish. Sprinkle almonds on top and bake uncovered for 15 min. at 350° F.

Yield: 4 servings

Crispy Baked Chicken

- 2 1/2-3 lb fryer, cut into pieces
- 1/2 c. milk or buttermilk
- 3/4 cup Seasoned Coating Mix (below)

Dip chicken pieces in milk, then Seasoned Coating Mix. Place chicken pieces, skin side up, in greased baking pan. Bake at 375° F until chicken is 165° in the center.

Seasoned Coating Mix

- 2 c. fine dry bread crumbs
- 2 T. onion powder
- 1 T. salt
- 2 t. poultry seasoning
- ½ t. garlic powder
- ½ t. paprika
- ½ t. dried thyme, crushed

Combine all ingredients and store in tightly covered container.

Dip chicken pieces, pork chops or fish fillets in milk, or beaten egg, then in coating mix. Shake off excess coating mix. Bake chicken or pork chops, covered, for 45 minutes at 350°. Remove cover and bake for an additional 15 minutes. Bake fish for 15-20 minutes at 350° F.

Yield: 2½ c. seasoned coating mix

Sweet and Sour Chicken

- 1 lb. boneless, skinless chicken breast
- 1 egg, beaten
- 1 T. water
- 2 T. butter or margarine
- ¼ c. cornstarch
- ¼ c. chicken broth
- 2 T. catsup
- ½ c. sugar
- ½ c. vinegar
- 1 T. soy sauce
- ½ t. salt
- 1 T. cornstarch or ThickGel®

Cut chicken into bite sized pieces. Combine beaten egg with water to make an egg wash. Dip chicken pieces into egg wash and dredge with cornstarch. Melt butter in heavy frying pan or spray pan well with pan spray and brown chicken pieces slowly over medium heat until well browned and juices are clear. Meanwhile, combine remaining ingredients in a small saucepan and bring to a boil over medium heat. Cook for 1 minute. Serve chicken pieces with sauce. This sauce is also an excellent when served with egg rolls or won tons.

Yield: 4 servings

Pineapple Chicken

- 2 T. olive oil
- 1 beaten egg
- 1 T. water
- 1 lb. chicken breast halves
- ¼ c. E-Z Gel® or flour

Sauce:

- 1 (20 oz.) can pineapple tidbits with juice
- 1 cup water
- ¼ c. sugar
- ¼ c. brown sugar
- 2 T. soy sauce
- 3 T. E-Z Gel®

Heat olive oil in heavy frying pan over medium high heat. Dip chicken pieces in egg wash made of beaten egg and water, then in E-Z Gel® (add salt, pepper or other seasonings for more flavor). Brown chicken on both sides in hot oil. Arrange in shallow baking pan and cover tightly with foil. Bake at 375 for 20 minutes (to an interior temp of 165 F). Meanwhile, combine pineapple tidbits, water, sugars and soy sauce in small saucepan over medium heat. Stir to dissolve sugar. Bring to a boil and add E-Z Gel®, stirring with a wire whisk. Pour over chicken pieces and serve with rice.

Yield: 4 servings

Seafood

Pan-fried Halibut

- 1 lb. halibut fillet
- 1 egg, slightly beaten
- 2 T. water
- ½ c. cornmeal
- ½ t. lemon-herb seasoning
- ½ t. salt
- ¼ t. pepper

Cut halibut fillet into serving size pieces. Combine egg and water in flat bowl. Combine cornmeal and seasonings in flat baking dish. Dip fillets into egg wash, then dredge with cornmeal mixture.

Heat 3 T. vegetable oil in frying pan over medium high heat. Add prepared fillets and cook until golden brown–about 5 minutes per side. Reduce heat and cook until fish is opaque and flakes easily with a fork.

Yield: 4 servings

Fish Fillets with Butter, Lemon, and Parsley

- ¼ c. flour
- 1 t. salt
- ¼ t. ground pepper
- 1 egg, slightly beaten
- 2 T. water
- 1 lb. trout, catfish, or other fish fillets
- 4 T. butter
- 1 T. vegetable oil
- 2 T. fresh lemon juice
- 1½ T. minced parsley

Combine flour, salt, and pepper in shallow pan. Combine egg and water in shallow bowl. Dip trout fillets in egg wash, then dredge in seasoned flour. Heat butter and oil in a heavy frying pan over medium heat until mixture sizzles. Add fish pieces and cook until golden brown–about 2 minutes per side. Remove cooked fish from pan, then stir in the lemon juice and cook until mixture is blended. Add the parsley, stir, and drizzle over cooked fillets. Serve immediately.

Yield: 4 servings

Oven-baked Halibut or Salmon

- 1 lb. halibut or salmon fillet
- 1 t. melted butter
- lemon-herb seasoning

Cut halibut fillet into serving size pieces. Place in shallow baking pan. Bake at 350° for 5 minutes. Drizzle with melted butter and sprinkle with seasoning. Continue baking until fish flakes easily with a fork. Do not over bake.

Yield: 4 servings

Hawaiian Sandwiches

- 1 can tuna fish, drained
- 1/4 c. Miracle Whip Salad Dressing
- 1-2 t. mustard
- 2 hamburger buns
- 4 pineapple rings, patted dry
- 4 large slices cheddar cheese

Preheat oven to 350°. Separate hamburger buns and lay all pieces out, crust side down, on a cookie sheet. Combine tuna, salad dressing, and mustard in a bowl. Divide tuna mix between the buns. Top with a circle of pineapple and a slice of cheese. Bake for 8-10 minutes until warmed through and cheese is toasty and bubbly.

Fish Tacos

- Halibut or tilapia
- 1-2 cups Panko Bread crumbs
- 1 large egg
- garlic salt
- lemon pepper
- 1 bag coleslaw mix (shredded cabbage and carrots.)
- lime wedges
- Cilantro lime dressing

In a shallow bowl whip egg with 1 tsp milk or water. In another shallow bowl combine bread crumbs and seasoning. Dredge fish in egg and then coat with bread crumbs. Fry in a shallow skillet in 1 Tbsp olive oil and 1 Tbsp butter until golden and flaky. Serve in warmed corn tortilla with coleslaw, drizzle dressing (or lime) on top.

Yield: 4 servings

Cilantro Lime Dressing

- 1/2 c. extra-virgin olive oil
- 1 jalapeno pepper, seeded and coarsely chopped
- 1 clove garlic, minced
- 3/4 t. minced ginger
- 1/4 c. lime juice

- 1/4 c. honey
- 2 t. balsamic vinegar
- 1/2 t. salt, or to taste
- 1/4 c. packed cilantro leaves

Mix in a blender until everything is mixed well. I also add a little Ultra Gel to thicken it slightly. Eat within 1 to 2 days.

Yield: 1 c.

Deep Fried Shrimp

- ½ c. flour
- 2 T. cornstarch or ThickGel®
- 1 t. baking powder
- ½ t. salt
- 1 egg
- Ice water
- 1 lb. jumbo shrimp, cleaned and deveined

Combine dry ingredients in a small bowl. Add egg and ice water to make a batter the consistency of thick cream. Stir well. Place at least 3" oil in deep fat fryer, wok, or frying pan and heat to 375°. Dip separate pieces of shrimp in prepared batter, then fry a few at a time until golden brown. If batter is too thin, it will fragment into the oil–add about 1 T. of flour to the batter and try again. Drain fried shrimp on a paper-towel lined plate to remove excess grease. Serve hot with cocktail or sweet and sour sauce.

Yield: 3-4 servings

Pan-fried Shrimp

- 1 lb. shrimp, peeled and deveined with tails removed
- ¼ c. butter
- 2 cloves garlic, minced
- 1 T. lemon or lime juice
- salt to taste

Prepare shrimp. Heat butter in heavy frying pan until melted and bubbly. Add garlic and sauté for a few seconds. Add one half of the shrimp, stirring constantly until the shrimp curl up and turn pink. Remove to serving plate. Repeat with remaining shrimp. Sprinkle with lemon or lime juice and season to taste.

Yield: 4 servings

Shrimp Alfredo

Prepare Pan-Fried Shrimp as directed. Fold into 4 c. prepared Alfredo sauce (Soups, Stews and Savory Sauces section) and serve over hot cooked and drained fettuccini noodles.

Side Dishes and Vegetables

Steamed Rice

Add ¼ t. salt to 2 c. water. Bring to a boil. Gradually add 1 c. rice, maintaining boil. Cover with a tight lid and reduce heat to low. Simmer for 20 minutes without removing the cover. Rice is done when water is completely absorbed and rice is tender. Fluff with a fork before serving.

*Double the cooking time and add 1/3 additional water for brown rice.

Yield: 4 servings

Baked Rice

Preheat oven to 400°. Combine 1 c. rice and ½ t. salt in a 2-quart casserole dish. Add 2 ½ c. boiling water. Cover tightly and bake for 30-45 minutes until water is absorbed and rice is tender.

*Double the cooking time for brown rice.

Yield: 4 servings

Ham Fried Rice with Vegetables

- 1 t. vegetable oil
- 1 T. chopped onion
- 2 T. chopped celery
- ½ c. finely chopped carrot
- ½ c. finely chopped ham
- 2 c. hot cooked rice
- 1 egg, slightly beaten
- 2 t. soy sauce
- 1 t. rice wine vinegar (opt)
- salt and pepper to taste

Heat oil in a wok or large sauté pan over medium high heat. Add onion, celery, carrot and ham; stir fry until vegetables are limp. Add rice and stir until mixture begins to brown. Push rice mixture to the side of the pan and add beaten egg, stirring until almost set, then combining with other ingredients. Stir in soy sauce, and vinegar, and season to taste.

Yield: 4 servings

Rice Pilaf

- 1 T. EACH vegetable oil and butter
- 1 c. long-grain rice
- ¼ c. chopped onion
- 1 clove garlic, crushed
- 2 c. water
- 1 t. chicken base
- 1 t. salt
- ¼ t. EACH dried thyme and sweet basil or herbs as desired

Melt together butter and vegetable oil over medium high heat. Add rice, onion, and garlic and cook, stirring constantly, until rice is golden brown. Add remaining ingredients. Reduce heat, cover and simmer for 20- 30 minutes until rice is tender.

Yield: 4 servings

Spanish Rice

- 2 T. olive oil
- ¼ c. chopped onion
- ¼ c. chopped green bell pepper (opt.)
- 2 cloves garlic, minced
- 1 serrano pepper, chopped fine (opt,)
- 1 cup long-grain rice
- ½ tsp salt
- ¼ tsp ground pepper
- 1 8-oz. can tomato sauce
- 1½ cups chicken broth

Heat oil in skillet over medium high heat. Add onion, green pepper, garlic, and rice and cook, stirring constantly, until rice is golden brown. Add remaining ingredients. Reduce heat, cover and simmer for 20-30 minutes until rice is tender.

Yield: 4 servings

"Funeral" Potatoes

- 2 (10¾-oz.) cans condensed cream of mushroom OR cream of chicken soup
- ¼ c. butter or margarine, melted
- 1 c. sour cream
- 2 T. dehydrated minced onion OR ¼ c. finely chopped onion
- 1 t. dried parsley
- 1 c. grated cheese
- 2 24-oz. bags frozen shredded hashbrown potatoes OR 6 russet potatoes, cooked, cooled and shredded
- ½ c. cornflakes, crushed
- 1 T. butter or margarine, melted

Combine first six ingredients in large bowl. Gently stir in potatoes to combine. Turn into 9" x 13" baking pan or 12" square casserole dish. Combine crushed cornflakes with 1 T. melted butter. Sprinkle over prepared potatoes. Bake uncovered in preheated 375° oven for about 1 hour until topping crisps and potatoes are bubbly

Yield: 12 servings

Herb-Baked Potatoes

- 4 medium potatoes
- 2 T. olive oil
- ½-1 t. dried herbs (oregano, thyme, rosemary, etc.)
- Kosher salt
- Ground pepper to taste

Preheat oven to 400°.Wash potatoes and cut into 1" cubes. Place olive oil in large baking sheet, add potatoes and turn over until all sides are well oiled. Sprinkle with herbs and seasonings. Bake for 20 minutes until potatoes are crispy on the outside and tender on the inside.

Yield: 4-6 servings

Everyday Mashed Potatoes

- 6 medium potatoes (russet, red, or Yukon gold)
- 1 t. salt
- ½ c. milk or cream
- 2 T. butter or margarine
- ½ c. sour cream (opt, particularly good with red potatoes)
- salt and pepper to taste

Peel potatoes and cut into uniform pieces. Add to medium saucepan and cover potatoes with water and 1 t. salt. Cook over high heat until water boils, then reduce heat to medium. Cover with a tight-fitting lid and cook for 20-30 minutes until potatoes are tender. Drain water and place potatoes in medium bowl with milk, butter, and sour cream. Mash with potato masher or whip on medium speed with electric mixer until smooth. Add additional milk and butter for desired consistency and season to taste.

Yield: 6 servings

Roasted Smashed Potatoes

6 medium Yukon gold potatoes

- ¼ c. olive oil
- 2 t. Kosher salt
- 1 t. finely chopped rosemary
- ½ t. onion powder
- ½ t. garlic powder
- ¼ t. paprika
- ¼ t. coarse ground black pepper

Place potatoes on foil-lined baking sheet. Pour 1 T. of the olive oil over the potatoes and rub with hands to coat. Sprinkle with Kosher salt and bake in preheated 350° oven for 45 minutes until potatoes are tender. Remove from the oven and cool for 10 minutes. Smash the potatoes with a flat dish or potato masher to ½" thickness. Pour remaining olive oil over the smashed potatoes and sprinkle with desired seasonings. Return to the hot oven and cook an additional 30-35 minutes until the potatoes are crispy.

Yield: 6 servings

Scalloped Potatoes

- 2 T. butter
- 2 T. flour
- 2 c. milk
- 1 ½ t. salt
- ½ t. pepper
- 4 medium potatoes, thinly sliced (golds are great for this)
- 2 T. chopped onion
- ½ c. grated cheddar cheese

Melt butter over medium heat in a large frying pan. Add flour and cook until bubbly and light tan, approximately 3 minutes. Add milk all at once and stir until thickened. Season with salt and pepper. Place half of the potatoes in a greased 2-quart casserole dish. Cover with half the onion and half the sauce. Repeat layers. Cover and bake at 350° for about 1 hour. Uncover, sprinkle with grated cheese, and bake 15 minutes longer.

Yield: 4 servings

Vegetable Stir Fry

Prepare vegetables as desired for stir fry:

- Carrots: Wash, peel and cut into ¼" slices or julienne strips.
- Celery: Wash and cut diagonally into ¼-½" slices.
- Broccoli : Wash and remove tough stem; peel and slice remaining stem into ¼" slices and break florets into bite-sized pieces.

- Cauliflower: Wash and break florets into bite-sized pieces.
- Peppers: Wash and remove stem end, seeds, and white membrane. Cut into ¼" thick slices.
- Snow Peas: Wash and remove stem ends and tough strings,
- Bulb Onion: Wash, peel and remove root and stem end. Dice.
- Green Onion: Wash and remove root ends and discard with outer layers as needed. Cut into ¼" slices up to green stem. Cut stems into ½" pieces.
- Bean Sprouts: Wash and remove wilted pieces.
- Mushrooms: Wash and cut into ¼" slices.
- Zucchini: Wash and remove stem and blossom end. Cut into ¼" slices.
- Garlic: Mince finely with a sharp knife or garlic press.
- Ginger Root: Peel and grate finely.

Heat 1-2 T. vegetable oil in heavy wok or sauté pan until very hot, but not smoking. Add garlic and ginger (if desired) to oil and cook for about 10 seconds. Add remaining vegetables, beginning with dense vegetables like carrots and cauliflower. Toss and stir vegetables to cook all surfaces. Add about 1 T. water. Cover with tight fitting lid and cook for 1-2 minutes until crisp-tender. Add ¼-½ c. water or broth and season to taste with soy sauce and spices. Combine 1 t. cornstarch with 2 T. cold water. Move vegetables to the side of the pan and add cornstarch mixture to the broth, stirring constantly until it boils and thickens to make a sauce. Add additional liquid or thickener, if necessary, for desired consistency.

Yield: 2 servings

Fresh Salsa

- 4 cups tomatoes, chopped
- 1 7-oz. can chopped green chilies
- 1-2 finely chopped, bell peppers
- 1-2 finely dice serrano peppers (opt.)
- 1 medium onion, peeled and grated
- ½ c. red wine vinegar
- 2 T. E-Z Gel®
- ½ T. ground cumin
- 1 T. chili powder
- 1/4 t. garlic powder
- 1 ½ t. salt
- 1 T. sugar

Combine chopped vegetables. Stir in remaining ingredients. Adjust seasonings to taste, adding a few drops tabasco sauce for a more spicy salsa. Store in a covered container in the refrigerator for up to one week or divide into freezer safe containers and freeze for up to three months.

Yield: about 6 cups

Quick Breads

Basic Muffins

- 1 c. flour
- 1½ t. baking powder
- ¼ t. salt
- 1 T. sugar
- 1 egg
- ½ c. milk
- 2 T. melted butter

Preheat oven to 375°. Combine dry ingredients. Combine egg, milk, and melted butter in another bowl. Add liquids to dry ingredients, stirring just to dampen dry ingredients. Spoon into greased muffin tins, filling 2/3 full. Bake for 20-25 minutes until golden brown and tests done.

Yield: 6 muffins

Poppy Seed Muffins

- 1 egg, beaten
- ¼ t. vanilla
- ¼ t. almond extract
- ¼ c. sugar
- 2 T. vegetable oil
- 2 T. applesauce
- 6 T. buttermilk or soured milk
- 2/3 c. flour
- 2 T. E-Z Gel®
- ½ t. soda
- ¼ t. salt
- 2 t. poppy seeds

Preheat oven to 350°. Combine egg, vanilla, almond extract and sugar and beat until smooth and lemon colored. Add oil, applesauce, and buttermilk and mix well. Combine flour, E-Z Gel®, soda, and salt and mix thoroughly. Add to creamed mixture. Stir in poppy seeds and spoon into prepared muffin tins, filling each cup 2/3 full. Bake until lightly brown–about 20 minutes.

Yield: 6-8 muffins.

Muffin Variations

Lemon Muffins: Prepare Poppy Seed Muffins as directed, substituting ½ t. finely grated lemon zest and ½ t. lemon extract for almond extract.

Orange Muffins: Prepare Poppy Seed Muffins as directed, substituting ½ t. finely grated orange zest and ½ t. orange extract for almond extract.

Chocolate Muffins: Prepare Poppy Seed Muffins as directed, omitting almond extract and poppy seeds. Add 2 T. cocoa to flour mixture. Add ¼ c. miniature chocolate chips if desired.

Blueberry Muffins: Prepare Poppy Seed Muffins as directed. Omit poppy seeds. Substitute ¼ teaspoon finely grated lemon zest and ¼ teaspoon lemon extract for almond extract. Fold in ½ cup canned or frozen blueberries (rinsed) before baking.

Banana-Chocolate Chip Muffins

- ¼ c. shortening or butter
- ¼ c. sugar
- 1 egg
- 1 t. vanilla
- ½ c. flour
- ¼ t. baking powder
- ¼ t. baking soda
- ¼ t. salt
- 1/3 c. mashed banana
- ¼ c. buttermilk or soured milk
- ¼ c. semi-sweet chocolate chips

Preheat oven to 350°. Beat shortening, sugar, egg and vanilla until fluffy. Add banana and buttermilk. Stir in dry ingredients until blended. Fold in chocolate chips. Fill greased and floured muffin tins 2/3 full. Bake 20-30 minutes until muffins test done. Let cool for 5 minutes, then remove from pans. Cool completely. If desired, frost with Cream Cheese Frosting.

Yield: 6 muffins

Apple Nut Muffins

- ½ c. flour
- ¼ t. soda
- ¼ t. salt
- ½ t. cinnamon
- ¼ t. nutmeg
- ¼ c. vegetable oil
- ¼ c. sugar
- 1 egg
- ½ t. vanilla
- ¼ c. milk
- ¾ c. peeled, grated cooking apple
- ¼ c. nuts (opt.)
- 2 T. cinnamon sugar (opt.)

Preheat oven to 350°. Combine dry ingredients and set aside. Beat together oil, sugar, egg and vanilla until light colored. Fold in milk, apples, and nuts. Add dry ingredients and stir until blended. Fill greased and floured muffin tins 1/2 full. If desired, sprinkle with cinnamon sugar. Bake for about 25 minutes until light brown. Cool for 5 minutes, then remove from tins and cool completely.

Yield: 6-8 muffins

Cinnamon Sugar Muffins

- ½ c. all-purpose flour
- ½ c. quick cooking rolled oats
- 1/3 c. packed brown sugar
- 1 t. baking powder
- 1 egg
- 2 T. vegetable oil
- 1/3 c. milk
- 2 T. brown sugar (reserve)
- ¼ t. ground cinnamon (reserve)

Preheat oven to 350° F. Combine first four ingredients. Combine egg, oil, and milk in another bowl. Add liquids to dry ingredients, mixing just until moistened (mixture will be lumpy). Fill greased muffin tins 2/3 full of batter. Sprinkle with mixture of 2 T. brown sugar and ¼ t. ground cinnamon. Bake 15-18 minutes.

Yield: 6 muffins

Nutty Coconut Muffins

- ½ c. sugar
- ¼ c. vegetable oil
- 1 egg, slightly beaten
- ½ t. coconut flavoring
- ¾ c. flour
- 1/8 t. baking soda
- 1/8 t. baking powder
- 1/8 t. salt
- ¼ c. buttermilk or soured milk
- ¼ c. flaked coconut
- ¼ c. chopped walnuts (opt.)

Cream together sugar, oil, egg, and flavoring in medium bowl. Sift together dry ingredients. Alternately add dry ingredients and buttermilk to make a thick batter. Fold in remaining ingredients and spoon into paper-lined muffin tins (2/3 full) or loaf pan. Bake muffins at 350° for 10-15 minutes until golden brown. Bake loaf at 325° F for about 30 minutes.

Meanwhile, combine ¼ c. sugar, 2 T. water, and 2 t. butter in small saucepan. Simmer gently for five minutes. Remove from heat and add ½ t. coconut flavoring. Prick small holes in top of baked bread with toothpick, then pour over hot syrup. Cool.

Yield: 8 muffins or 1 medium loaf

Lemon Muffins

- ¼ c. softened butter
- ½ c. sugar
- 1 T. lemon juice
- 1 egg
- ¾ c. flour
- ¾ t. baking powder
- ¼ t. salt
- ¼ c. milk
- ½ t. finely grated lemon zest

Cream together butter, sugar, lemon juice and egg in medium bowl. Sift together dry ingredients. Alternately add dry ingredients and milk to make a thick batter. Stir in lemon zest. Spoon into paper-lined muffin tins (1/2 full) or loaf pan. Bake muffins at 350° for 10-15 minutes until golden brown. Bake loaf at 325° F for about 30 minutes.

Meanwhile, combine 2 T. lemon juice and ¼ c. sugar in medium saucepan. Heat just until sugar is dissolved. Prick small holes in top of baked bread with toothpick, then gently pour lemon syrup into holes. Cool.

Yield: 8 muffins or 1 medium loaf

Corn Bread

- 1/3 c. sugar
- 1/3 c. vegetable oil
- 3 eggs
- 1 t. vanilla
- 2 c. buttermilk OR 2 c. soured milk
- 1 c. cornmeal
- 1 ¼ c. flour
- 1 t. soda
- ½ t. salt

Preheat oven to 375°. Combine sugar, oil, eggs and vanilla and beat until smooth and lemon colored. Add buttermilk and mix well. Combine dry ingredients, then add to batter, mixing thoroughly. Pour into greased and floured 9" x 13" pan. Bake for 30-40 minutes until lightly browned and tests done. Cool for 10 minutes before cutting. Serve with honey butter.

Yield: 12 servings

Lemon Bread

- ¼ c. butter
- ½ c. sugar
- 1 T. lemon juice
- 1 egg
- ¾ c. flour
- ¾ t. baking powder
- ¼ t. salt
- ¼ c. milk
- ½ t. finely grated lemon zest

Cream together butter, sugar, lemon juice, and egg in medium bowl. Sift together dry ingredients. Alternately add dry ingredients and milk to creamed mixture to make a thick batter. Stir in lemon zest. Spoon into paper-lined and lightly greased loaf pan. Bake loaf at 325 degrees for about 30-45 minutes until edges are brown and center tests done.

Meanwhile, combine 2 T. lemon juice and 1/4 c. sugar in medium saucepan. Heat just until sugar is dissolved. Prick small holes in top of baked bread with toothpick. Pour glaze over loaf and cool.

Banana Bread

- 2 c. flour
- 1 t. baking soda
- ½ t. salt
- 1 t. cinnamon
- ½ c. butter, softened
- ½ c. brown sugar
- ¼ c. sugar
- 2 eggs
- 1 t. vanilla
- 1 ¼ c. mashed over ripe bananas

Preheat oven to 350 degrees F. Grease and flour an 8x4 inch loaf pan.

In a small bowl combine flour, baking soda, salt, and cinnamon. In a medium bowl combine butter, brown sugar, and white sugar and beat well. Add the eggs and vanilla and mix. Scrape down the side of the bowl. Stir in mashed bananas. Add the dry ingredients and stir just until combined. Do not over mix!

Pour the batter into the prepared loaf pan and bake for 50-60 minutes or until center tests clean.

Cool in the pan for 5 minutes. Remove and cool completely before eating.

Yield: 1 loaf

Sour Cream Coffee Cake

- ½ c. softened butter
- ½ c. sugar
- 2 eggs
- ½ c. sour cream
- 1¼ c. cake flour
- 1 t. baking powder
- ½ t. baking soda
- ¼ t. salt
- 1 t. grated lemon zest
- ½ c. milk

Filling and Topping:

- ¼ c. brown sugar
- 1 t. cinnamon

Preheat oven to 350°. Combine butter, sugar, eggs and sour cream and beat well. Combine dry ingredients and add to sour cream mixture. Fold in lemon. Gradually add milk to make a smooth batter.

Combine ingredients for filling. Spread half of the batter in a greased and floured 8" x 8" baking pan. Sprinkle with half of the filling. Spread with remaining batter and filling. Bake for 25 to 30 minutes until tests done.

Yield: 12 servings

Pancakes

- 2 c. flour
- 3 T. sugar
- 2 ½ t. baking powder
- ½ t. salt
- 1 egg
- 3 T. oil
- 1 ½ c. milk

In a large mixing bowl, combine flour, sugar, baking powder, and salt and mix well. Combine egg, oil, and milk and stir well. Add wet mixture to dry, stirring just enough to bring together. There may still be a few lumps, that's okay. Add additional milk if needed. Heat an electric griddle to 400 degrees. Grease lightly. Scoop batter into circles on griddle. Cook on both sides until browned and done through. Serve with maple syrup, jam, or whipping cream!

Yield: 4-6 servings

Baking Powder Biscuits

- 1¾ c. all-purpose flour
- 1/3 c. cake flour
- ½ t. salt
- 1 T. baking powder
- 1 T. sugar
- ½ c. vegetable shortening
- ¾ c. milk

Preheat oven to 425°. Combine dry ingredients in medium bowl. Cut in shortening until mixture resembles coarse meal. Add milk all at once and stir just until dough forms a ball. Turn the dough onto a lightly floured board and knead 12 times. Pat or roll ½" thick. Cut into rounds with 2" cutter. Bake on greased baking sheet for 15-20 minutes until golden brown and flaky.

Yield: 8 biscuits

Buttermilk Biscuits

Prepare Baking Powder Biscuits or E-Z Gel® Baking Powder Biscuits as directed, substituting buttermilk or sour milk for milk. Reduce baking powder to 1½ t. and add ½ t. soda.

Cheese Biscuits

Prepare Baking Powder Biscuits or E-Z Gel® Baking Powder Biscuits as directed. Add ½ c. grated cheddar cheese to the dry ingredients.

E-Z Gel® Baking Powder Biscuits

Really tender and moist

- 1 2/3 c. all purpose flour
- 1/3 c. cake flour
- 2 T. E-Z Gel® modified food starch
- 1 T. baking powder
- ½ t. salt
- 1 T. sugar
- ½ c. shortening
- 2/3 c. milk

Preheat oven to 425°. Combine dry ingredients. Cut in shortening until mixture resembles coarse meal. Add the milk all at once and let stand for 1 minute. Stir just until the dough forms a ball around the fork. Turn the dough onto a lightly floured board and knead about 12 times to form a very soft dough. Pat or roll ½-¾" thick. Cut into rounds. Place on ungreased baking sheet and bake for 12-15 minutes until golden brown and flaky.

Yield: 8 biscuits

Quick Fry Bread

- 2 c. white or wheat flour
- 1 T. baking powder
- 1 t. salt
- 1 c. hot water
- 1 T. vegetable oil

Combine dry ingredients in a medium bowl. Add hot water and oil to make a soft dough. Knead on lightly floured board. Divide into 16 pieces and roll thin. Fry in ½" of hot oil. Serve with honey butter.

Yield: 8 servings

Honey Butter

- 1 c. butter, softened
- 3 T. honey, soft but not hot

In a small bowl whip butter with an electric mixer until light and fluffy. Fold in honey until fully incorporated. Store in the refrigerator.

Yield: 1 1/2 cups

Sopapillas

- 2 c. flour
- 1 t. baking powder
- 1 t. salt
- 1 egg
- 3 T. vegetable oil
- ½ c. water

Combine egg, oil, and water and add to dry ingredients. Knead until smooth. Divide into two parts and roll each into a 12-inch square. Cut into 3-inch squares (16). Fry in 2 inches of oil (preheated to 375°) for 3-4 minutes, turning when golden brown. Drain well and sprinkle with powdered sugar.

Yield: 32 Sopapillas

Peanut Butter Marshmallow Spread

- 1 c. creamy peanut butter
- 1 c. marshmallow creme
- 1 t. honey if needed to thin mix

Whip together peanut butter and marshmallow creme. Add warm honey or a splash of milk if the mixture is too thick. Serve on hot Sopapillas or Fry bread. Never think about the calorie count. It's delicious.

Yield: 2 cups

Bread Sticks

- 2 c. flour
- 2 T. sugar
- 1 ½ t. baking powder
- 1 t. salt
- 2 T. olive oil
- 2/3 c. milk
- ¼ c. Parmesan cheese
- ½ t. garlic powder
- ½ t. dried parsley
- 1 t. sesame seeds

Combine dry ingredients in medium bowl. Add oil and milk and mix until dough clings together. Knead 10-12 times on floured surface. Roll into an 8" square. Cut into strips. Place on greased baking sheet and brush with melted butter. Combine Parmesan cheese, garlic powder, parsley and sesame seeds in small bowl. Sprinkle breadsticks with cheese mixture and bake at 400° for 10-15 minutes until golden brown.

Yield: 1 dozen

Flour Tortillas

- 2 c. flour
- ¾ t. salt
- ¾ t. baking powder
- 2 T. vegetable oil
- ½ - ¾ c. hot water (120-140° F)

Combine dry ingredients. Add oil and work with hands until oil particles are dispersed. Add water, stirring with hands to make a soft dough. Divide into 1" balls. Flatten, cover with plastic wrap, and let stand for 10 minutes. Roll on floured surface until very thin and 8-10" in diameter. Cook on ungreased frying pan or griddle over medium heat until brown spots appear, about 30 seconds. Repeat on other side.

Yield: 1 dozen

Yeast Breads and Rolls

Basic Bread for High Altitudes

- 6 T. sugar
- 6 T. shortening
- 2 T. salt
- 5 c. scalded milk
- 1 T. dry yeast dissolved in
- ½ c. warm water
- 10-12 c. bread flour

Combine sugar, shortening, salt and scalded milk in large bowl. Add 6 c. flour and mix thoroughly with electric mixer. Stir in dissolved yeast and beat an additional 2-4 minutes. Add flour to make a soft dough. Knead well. Let rise until double (2-3 hours). Shape into four loaves and let rise until double (1-1½ hours), then bake at 375° for 30-40 minutes. Brush with butter or shortening after removing from the oven for a soft, chewy crust.

Yield: 4 loaves

Freezer White Bread

- 5- 6 c. bread flour
- 3 T. dry yeast
- 2 c. very hot tap water (120°)
- 4 T. sugar
- 2 T. shortening
- 2 t. salt

Combine 2 c. flour and yeast in a large mixing bowl. Add 2 c. very hot tap water (120°), sugar, shortening, and salt and mix thoroughly with electric mixer. Add flour to make a soft dough. Knead well. Let rise until double (about 1 hour). Divide in half and shape into loaves. Wrap tightly and freeze for up to six months. To bake, place in greased loaf pans and let thaw at room temperature until double (about 3 hours). Bake at 375° for 30-40 minutes. Brush with butter or shortening after removing from the oven for a soft, chewy crust. Also works well for pizza crust.

Yield: 2 loaves

Foolproof Wheat Bread

- 1 T. yeast dissolved in ¼ c. warm water
- 2½ c. hottest tap water
- 2 c. whole wheat flour
- 2 T. vital wheat gluten
- 3 T. vegetable oil
- 3 T. honey
- 3 T. molasses
- 1 T. salt
- 2-4 c. additional wheat flour

Dissolve yeast in ¼ c. warm water. Combine 2½ c. hot water, 2 c. flour, and gluten in large mixing bowl. Add oil, honey, molasses, and salt. Beat well with electric mixer. Stir in dissolved yeast and additional flour to make a soft dough. Knead well (8-10 minutes). Divide into two portions and shape each into a loaf. Place in greased loaf tins, lightly grease top of each loaf, and let rise until not quite double. Bake at 350° for30-40 minutes until golden brown. Remove bread from pans immediately. Brush crust with shortening or butter and cover with a towel to cool.

Yield: 2 large loaves

Quick Rise Bread Sticks

- 1 c. warm water
- 1 T. yeast
- 1 T. sugar
- 2 T. olive oil
- 1 t. salt
- 2-3 c. bread flour

Dissolve yeast and sugar in warm water. Add olive oil, salt and flour and knead until smooth and elastic. Let rest for 10-15 minutes. Shape into bread sticks and place on greased baking sheet. Brush with melted butter and a mixture of ¼ c. Parmesan cheese, ½ t. garlic salt, and 1 t. dried parsley. Let rise 10 minutes. Bake at 375° F for 20 minutes or until golden brown.

Yield: 16 bread sticks

French Bread

- 3 c. warm water
- 2 T. yeast
- 1 c. scalded milk, cooled
- 5 T. shortening
- 4 T. sugar
- 1 T. salt
- 7-9 c. bread flour

Dissolve yeast in warm water. Add milk, shortening, sugar, yeast, salt and 4 c. flour. Beat well with electric mixer. Add additional flour to make a soft dough. Knead well. Let rise until double (about 2 hours). Divide into three portions and shape each into a long roll. Place onto a baking sheet which has been sprinkled with cornmeal. Slash each loaf four or five times diagonally with a sharp knife and brush with a mixture of 1 beaten egg and 1 t. salt. Sprinkle with sesame seeds, let rise, and bake at 375° for about 45 minutes or until golden brown.

Yield: 3 loaves

Bread Bowls

- 2 T. yeast
- 4 c. warm water
- ¼ c. sugar
- 1½ t. salt
- ¼ c. shortening or vegetable oil
- 7-9 c. bread flour

Dissolve yeast in water. Add sugar, salt, shortening, and 4 c. flour. Beat well with electric mixer. Add additional flour to make a soft dough. Knead well. Cover and let rise about 1 hour. Form into balls approximately the size of baseballs. Place on greased baking sheet. Let rise until double, about 45 minutes. Bake at 400° for 15-20 minutes until golden brown. Cool on rack. To serve, cut small slice off the top of each loaf. Scoop out the soft bread from the inside, leaving a ½" thick shell. Fill with thick soup and serve with the bread that was removed from the inside of the bowl.

Yield: 10-12 medium bowls

Pain Ordinaire

Authentic French Bread

- ½ T. dry yeast
- 1 t. sugar
- 2 c. warm water
- 2 t. salt
- 5-6 c. bread flour

Add yeast and sugar to warm water. Let stand until foamy (10 minutes). Add 2 c. flour and salt; beat well with electric mixer. Add additional flour to make a stiff dough. Knead well. Dough will become soft and pliable after sufficient kneading. Return dough to bowl and let rise until double in bulk (about 2 hours). Punch down and let rise again until double in bulk (about 1 ½ hours). Shape into two large loaves, 4 small loaves or 36 buns (may also be used for the world's best pizza dough after the first rising; makes two 16-inch pizzas). Combine 1 egg white, 1 T. water and a pinch of salt to make egg wash. Brush on loaves or buns. Slash large loaves 4-5 times with a sharp knife or razor blade and sprinkle with sesame seeds. Let rise for 30 minutes. Bake 25-30 minutes at 400° F to a rich golden brown.

Yield: 2 large loaves or 36 buns

Bea's Buttermilk Rolls

- 1 c. buttermilk
- ¼ t. baking soda
- 1 t. salt
- 3 T. sugar
- 3 T. shortening
- 1 T. yeast dissolved in
- ½ c. water
- 2½-3½ c. flour

Heat buttermilk to lukewarm. Add soda, sugar, and shortening. Beat well and add 1 c. flour. Add dissolved yeast, ½ c. flour, and salt. Add remaining flour as needed to make a soft dough. Let rise until double. Shape into rolls and let rise until double. Bake at 400° for 10-20 minutes.

Yield: 2 dozen rolls

Fanfare French Twists

- 3 c. warm water
- 1 t. sugar
- 1 T. dry yeast
- 3 T. shortening
- 1 t. onion salt
- 2 t. salt
- 2 egg yolks
- about 7 c. bread flour
- cornmeal
- 2 egg whites
- ½ t. salt
- sesame of poppy seeds

Dissolve sugar and yeast in warm water. Add shortening, onion salt, salt, and 3 c. flour. Beat well with electric mixer (3-5 minutes). Stir in egg yolks and additional flour to make a stiff dough. Knead well. Let rise until double (about 2 hours). Punch down and let rise again (about 1 hour). Shape into rolls and place on baking sheets which have been sprinkled with corn meal. Beat egg whites and ½ t. salt until frothy. Brush tops of rolls with egg white mixture and sprinkle with seeds. Let rise until double (about ½ hour). Bake for 15-20 minutes at 400° until golden brown.

Yield: 3 dozen rolls

Sixty Minute Rolls

- ½ c. cold water
- 1 c. scalded milk
- 2 T. yeast
- ¼ c. margarine or butter
- 3 T. sugar
- 1 t. salt
- 3½-4 c. bread flour

Combine water and milk in large bowl. Add yeast, margarine, sugar, salt and 2 c. flour and beat well with electric mixer. Stir in additional flour to make a soft dough. Knead well. Let rest for 10 minutes then shape as desired. Let rise until double (about 30 minutes). Bake at 400° for 10-15 minutes or until golden brown.

Yield: 3 dozen rolls

Hard Rolls

- 1 c. warm water
- 1 T. yeast
- 1 T. sugar
- 1 t. salt
- 2 T. olive oil or shortening
- 3 ½-4 c. bread flour
- 2 egg whites, slightly beaten (reserve 1 T.)

Combine water, yeast, sugar, salt, oil, and about half of the flour. Beat well. Add egg whites (except reserved 1 T.) and beat well. Add flour to form a soft dough. Knead well. Let rise until double. Punch down and let rise again. Form balls about 1½ inches in diameter and place about 4 inches apart on a greased or parchment lined baking sheet. Let rise until double. Brush with reserved egg white and sprinkle with sesame seeds or poppy seeds if desired. Place a 9" x 13" pan half filled with boiling water on bottom rack of oven for crusty rolls. Bake at 400° for 20 minutes or until golden brown.

Yield: 2 dozen rolls

Hamburger Buns

- 2 T. yeast
- 4½ c. warm water
- 1 c. dry milk
- ½ c. shortening
- ½ c. sugar
- 2 T. salt
- 2 eggs
- 10-12 c. bread flour

Dissolve yeast in warm water. Add dry milk, shortening, sugar, salt, and 5 c. flour and beat well with electric mixer. Add eggs and beat again. Stir in additional flour to make a soft dough. Let rise until double. Punch down and let rise again. Roll out to ½" thickness. Cut into hamburger buns with a large bottle ring. Place on greased baking sheet and let rest 5 minutes. Press each bun down lightly with hand, then brush tops with beaten egg white. Let rise until double and bake at 400° for 12-15 minutes until golden brown.

Yield: 4 dozen

Basic Sweet and Dinner Rolls

- ½ c. warm water
- 2 T. yeast
- 2 c. scalded milk, cooled for 5 minutes
- ¼-½ c. sugar
- ¼-½ c. shortening
- 2 t. salt
- 2 eggs
- 5-6 c. bread flour

Dissolve yeast in warm water. Set aside. Combine scalded milk, sugar, shortening, and salt with 3 c. flour. Beat until smooth. Beat in eggs and dissolved yeast, then add additional flour to make a soft dough. Knead well. Let rise until double (30-45 minutes). Shape as desired. Let rise again. Bake dinner rolls at 400° for 10-15 minutes, fruit-filled sweet rolls at 350° for 25-30 minutes, and filled sweet rolls (other than fruit-filled) at 375° for 20-30 minutes. Glaze with powdered sugar glaze if desired.

Yield: 4 dozen dinner rolls OR 4 large sweet rolls

Freezer Sweet Rolls

- 1¼ c. flour
- 1 t. salt
- 2 T. yeast
- ¾ c. sugar
- ½ c. margarine
- 1 c. very hot tap water (120°)
- 2 eggs
- 1-2 c. flour

Combine 1 ¼ c. flour, salt, yeast, sugar, margarine, and water in large mixing bowl. Beat with electric mixer for 3 minutes. Add eggs and beat an additional 1 minute. Stir in flour to make a soft dough. Knead well. Shape as desired. Wrap and freeze for up to 6 weeks. To bake, remove from freezer and arrange on greased baking sheet. Let thaw and rise until double (about 3 hours). Bake at 375° until golden brown. HINT: Small rolls thaw and rise more evenly than very large ones. Fruit fillings require more time to thaw than sugar fillings.

Yield: 2 medium rolls or 2 dozen small rolls

Refrigerator Orange Rolls

- 1 c. evaporated milk
- 1 c. very hot tap water (120°)
- 1 c. sugar
- ½ c. softened butter
- 2 t. salt
- 6 eggs
- 2 T. yeast
- 2 T. sugar
- ½ c. warm water
- 7-8 c. bread flour

Combine milk, 1 c. hot water, 1 c. sugar, butter, salt and eggs. Dissolve yeast and 2 T. sugar in warm water and add to the milk mixture. Gradually add flour and beat well. DO NOT KNEAD! Let rise until double. Refrigerate overnight, or up to five days. Divide into four portions. Roll each into an oblong rectangle. Spread with margarine and sprinkle with orange sugar. Roll like cinnamon rolls and seal well. Cut into 1" slices. Place in well-greased muffin tins and let rise 1 hour. Bake at 400° for 8 minutes. Do not over bake. Tip upside down on waxed paper so the sugar runs to the top. Cool slightly, then turn upright.

Yield: 75 rolls

Orange Sugar

- 2 c. sugar
- grated zest of one orange
- 1 T. orange extract

Combine ingredients in a small bowl or blend in a blender or food processor until well mixed. Place remaining sugar in airtight container and refrigerate for use at a later time.

Yield: 2 cups

Orange Filling

Combine 6 T. butter, 1 c. sugar, and the grated rind of 1 orange (or 1-2 T. orange juice concentrate) in a small sauce pan. For a more syrupy filling, add 1-2 T. light corn syrup. Cook filling over medium heat to desired consistency.

Yield: 1 cup

Orange Glaze

Add 1 T. melted margarine and 2-4 T. orange juice to 1 c. powdered sugar to make desired consistency.

Yield: ½ cup

Powdered Sugar Glaze

Combine 2 c. powdered sugar, 2-3 T. softened or melted butter or margarine, and about ¼ c. hot milk or water. Blend well. Add ½ t. vanilla or other extract and adjust liquid for desired consistency. Glaze rolls either hot or after they have cooled.

Yield: 1½ cup

Crumb Topping

- 1/3 c. flour
- 1 t. cinnamon
- 1/3 c. brown sugar
- 2 T. butter

Combine dry ingredients. Cut in butter with a fork until blended. Sprinkle over sweet rolls before baking and eliminate the glaze. Especially good on fruit-filled rolls.

Yield: ¾ cup

Caramel for Pecan Rolls

- ½ c. butter
- 1 c. brown sugar
- ½ c. light corn syrup
- 1 c. pecans or walnuts

Combine butter, brown sugar, and light corn syrup in saucepan over medium heat. Stir well. Boil until sugar dissolves, then add nuts if desired. Also works great for monkey bread, pull away rolls, or bubble loafs.

Yield: 2½ cups

Cherry Nut Filling

Drain 1 pint frozen, thawed pitted cherries. In blender, grind cherries with 1 t. lemon juice and 1/2 cup chopped nuts. In saucepan, blend cherry mixture with 2 T. cornstarch and 1/3 c. sugar. Bring to boil and cook until thick. If necessary, filling may be thinned with a little cherry juice to reach desired consistency.

Other Fun Fillings!

- Powdered flavored gelatin
- Jams and jellies
- Softened cream cheese mixed with mini chocolate chips

Spudnuts

- 2 c. scalded milk
- ½ c. sugar
- ½ c. shortening
- 2 t. salt
- ½ t. nutmeg
- ½ t. lemon extract
- 3 eggs
- 1 c. mashed potatoes
- 2 T. yeast dissolved in
- ½ c. warm water
- 5-6 c. bread flour

Combine milk, sugar, shortening, salt, nutmeg, lemon extract, and potatoes in a large bowl. Add 3 cups flour and beat well. Add softened yeast and eggs and beat an additional 2 minutes. Add flour to make a soft dough. Knead well. Let rise until double (about 1 hour). Roll out, cut and let rise slightly. Heat about 2" vegetable oil in heavy frying pan to 375°. Fry spudnuts in hot oil. Glaze and garnish as desired.

Yield: 3 dozen

Pocket Bread (Pita Bread)

- 1 c. warm water
- 1½ t. dry yeast
- 2 T. oil
- ¾ t. salt
- 2 c. flour
- 1 t. baking powder

Dissolve yeast in warm water. Add remaining ingredients and knead well, adding additional flour as necessary to make a soft dough. Let rest 15 minutes. Divide dough into 6 pieces. Cover with plastic wrap and let rest 10-15 minutes. Place dark metal baking sheet or pizza stone (follow manufacturer directions) in oven for 10 minutes to preheat at 450°. Flatten each dough ball with rolling pin to about ¼" thickness. Place on a preheated baking sheet or stone, two at a time, and bake until puffed and lightly browned. Cool. Fill as desired.

Yield: 10 pita breads

Wheat Pita Breads

- 1 T. yeast
- 1½ c. warm water
- ¼ c. honey
- 1 T. salt
- 2 T. olive oil
- 1 ½ c. bread flour
- 1 ½ c. whole wheat flour

Dissolve yeast in water. Add honey, salt and oil. Let stand 10 minutes. Combine flours in large mixing bowl. Gradually add liquid to flour mixture, working with hands to form a moist, flexible dough. Knead well, adding addition flour if necessary to form a soft dough. Let dough rest for 5 minutes, then divide into 18 pieces. Place dark metal baking sheet or pizza stone (follow manufacturer directions) in oven for 10 minutes to preheat at 450°. Flatten each dough ball with rolling pin to about ¼" thickness. Place on a baking sheet, two at a time, and bake at 450° until puffed and golden brown. Cool. Fill as desired.

Yield: 24 pita breads

English Muffins

- 1 c. milk
- 1 c. water
- 3 T. butter
- 4-5 c. bread flour
- 1 T. dry yeast
- 2 T. sugar
- 1 t. salt
- 2 T. cornmeal

Scald milk in medium saucepan. Remove from heat and add butter and water. Combine 3 c. flour, yeast, sugar, salt and warmed liquids in large mixing bowl. Beat well. Add additional flour to form a soft dough. Knead well. Place in greased bowl and let rise for 30 minutes. Punch down and roll to ½" thickness on canvas which has been sprinkled with cornmeal. Cut with floured 3-inch round cutter. Cover and let rise 30 minutes. Preheat lightly buttered griddle on medium low heat (approx. 250° F). Brown muffins 15-20 minutes on each side. Cool.

Yield: 18-20 muffins

Easy Refrigerator Croissants

- 4 c. flour
- 1 c. chilled butter
- 1 c. warm water
- 2 T. sugar
- 1 T. dry yeast
- 1½ t. salt
- ¾ c. evaporated milk
- 1 egg
- 1 c. flour
- ½ c. butter, melted
- 1 egg
- 2 T. evaporated milk

Cut butter into flour until size of kidney beans. Set aside in refrigerator. In large bowl, combine warm water and sugar; sprinkle yeast over mixture. Set aside to bubble for 5 minutes. Add salt, evaporated milk, 1 egg and 1 c. flour; beat on medium speed with mixer until smooth. Stir in melted butter. Pour yeast mixture over flour-butter mixture. Stir with wooden spoon to moisten flour. Cover bowl; chill for 2 hours or up to 1 week.

Three hours before serving, remove dough from bowl and knead very lightly. Divide dough into fourths. Roll each fourth into a 14-inch circle and cut into 8 or 12 wedges. Roll to form crescent and place on ungreased baking sheet with point tucked underneath. Let rise for 2 hours. Before baking, brush with egg wash made by beating together 1 egg and 2 T. evaporated milk. Bake at 375° for 15-20 minutes until golden brown. Cool.

Yield: 32-48 croissants

Soft Pretzels

- 3 T. yeast
- 4 c. warm water
- 1 t. sugar
- 2 T. salt
- 8-10 c. bread flour

Dissolve yeast and sugar in warm water and let stand 10 minutes. Add remaining ingredients to form a soft dough. Knead well. Place in greased bowl and let rise until double. Divide into 48 pieces. Shape each into a rope 18 inches long and twist into pretzel shape. Boil together 4 c. water and 4 t. baking soda. Drop one pretzel into boiling liquid until it floats, about 1 minute, remove, drain and place on baking sheet. Sprinkle with coarse salt. Repeat with remaining pretzels. Bake at 450° for 12 minutes until golden brown and shiny.

Yield: 48 large pretzels

Bagels

- 3 c. warm water
- 1 T. yeast
- 2 T. sugar
- 1 T. salt
- 8-9 c. bread flour
- 4 quarts water
- 1 T. sugar
- 1 egg white
- 1 T. cold water

Combine water, yeast, and sugar in large bowl. Set aside for 10 minutes until yeast foams. Add 3 c. flour and salt and beat with an electric mixer for 3 minutes. Add additional flour by hand to make a very stiff dough. Turn onto floured surface and knead well, adding flour as necessary. Place in greased bowl, cover with plastic wrap and let rise until double, about 1 hour. Divide dough into 16 pieces. Shape each piece into a smooth ball and let rest for five minutes. Flatten each ball slightly and poke a hole in each center, pulling with fingers to open a hole in the center about 1" in diameter. Place on a greased baking sheet, cover with plastic wrap and let rise for 30 minutes.

Combine 4 quarts water and 2 T. sugar in a large frying pan and bring to a gentle boil. Drop 3-4 bagels at a time into boiling liquid and simmer for 30 seconds to 1 minute on each side. Place cooked bagels on paper towels to remove excess water.

Combine egg white and cold water to make an egg wash. Place bagels on greased baking sheet and brush with egg wash. Top with sesame seeds, poppy seeds, dried onion, herbs, etc. as desired. Bake at 400° F. for 25-30 minutes until golden brown. Cool on wire racks.

Yield: 16 large bagels

Brownies, Bars, and Cookies

Brownies and Bars

Chocolate Marshmallow Brownie Bars

- 2 c. sugar
- 1 c. butter
- 1/3 c. cocoa powder
- 4 eggs
- 1 ½ c. flour

Mix all ingredients together in the order listed. Beat well. Transfer to a lightly greased 9x13 inch pan. Bake at 350° F for 30-45 minutes. Cover with 1 small package miniature marshmallows and bake 5 more minutes until marshmallows are puffed and melted. Cool and frost with chocolate icing.

Brownies

- 1 c. butter
- ¼ c. cocoa
- 2 c. flour
- 2 c. sugar
- 4 eggs

Preheat oven to 350° F. Grease and flour 9" x 13" baking pan. Melt butter in medium saucepan. Add cocoa. Meanwhile combine flour and sugar in medium bowl. Stir in butter/cocoa mixture, and then beat in eggs. Pour into prepared pan and bake for 30 minutes. Sprinkle with powdered sugar or ice with chocolate frosting before serving.

Yield: 2 dozen

Chocolate Icing

Combine ½ c. butter with ½ c. cocoa powder. Beat well with electric mixer. Add about ½ c. evaporated milk, ½ t. vanilla and 1 lb. or more powdered sugar for desired consistency.

Yield: 2 cups

Luscious Lemon Bars

Crust:

- 1 c. soft butter
- dash salt
- ½ c. powdered sugar
- 2 c. flour

Combine ingredients and mix well. Press mixture into 9" x 13" baking pan. Bake at 350° F. for 15 minutes or until golden brown.

Filling:

- 2 c. sugar
- 2 T. flour OR ¼ c. E-Z Gel®
- 6 T. lemon or lime juice
- 4 eggs, beaten

Combine sugar and flour in medium bowl. Combine eggs and lemon juice and stir into dry mixture. Pour onto slightly cooled crust and sprinkle with powdered sugar. Bake an additional 25 minutes.

Yield: 24 bars

Peanut Butter Fingers

- ½ c. butter
- ½ c. sugar
- ½ c. brown sugar
- 1 egg
- ½ t. vanilla
- 1/3 c. peanut butter
- ½ t. baking soda
- ¼ t. salt
- 1 c. flour
- 1 c. oats (quick or regular)

Cream together butter, sugars, egg, vanilla and peanut butter. Stir in dry ingredients. Spread into greased 9" x 13" baking pan and bake at 350° F. for 20-25 minutes until lightly browned. Cool slightly and frost with peanut butter frosting, chocolate frosting or both.

Yield: 2 dozen

Peanut Butter Frosting

Cream together ¼ c. butter or margarine, ¼ to ½ c. peanut butter and ¼ c. warm milk or cream. Beat in 1 lb. powdered sugar. Add additional milk or powdered sugar for desired consistency.

Cookies

Chocolate Chip Cookies

- 1 c. butter or margarine
- ¾ c. sugar
- ¾ c. brown sugar
- 2 eggs
- 2 t. vanilla
- 2⅓ c. flour
- 1 t. baking soda
- ½ t. salt
- 6 oz. chocolate chips

Preheat oven to 375°. Cream together butter and sugars on medium speed with electric mixer for 10 minutes. Mixture will be light tan and creamy. Add eggs and vanilla and continue beating until combined. Stir in dry ingredients and chocolate chips. Drop by tablespoons onto ungreased baking sheets. Bake for 9-11 minutes until light brown. Let stand for 3-4 minutes before removing from tray.

Yield: 2 dozen cookies

High Altitude: Add 2 teaspoons water to creamed mixture; increase flour to 2½ c.

Chocolate Cookies

- 2 c. flour
- ¾ t. baking soda
- ½ t. salt
- 1 c. butter
- 1 ½ c. sugar
- 2/3 c. cocoa powder
- 2 eggs
- 2 t. vanilla
- 1 c. chopped nuts (opt.)
- 2 c. chocolate, vanilla, or peanut butter chips

Preheat oven to 375°. Sift together dry ingredients and set aside.

Cream together butter and sugar in large bowl with electric mixer. Blend in cocoa and E-Z Gel®. Add eggs one at a time, beating after each addition. Mix in vanilla. Stir in dry ingredients, nuts and chocolate, vanilla or peanut butter chips. Drop by spoonsful onto ungreased baking sheets. Bake at 350° for 8-10 minutes. DO NOT OVERBAKE!

Cool for 5 minutes on baking sheet. Transfer cookies to rack and cool completely. Store in airtight container or freeze.

Yield: 3 dozen

Peanut Butter Cookies

- ½ c. butter, softened
- ½ c. peanut butter
- ½ c. granulated sugar
- ½ c. brown sugar
- ¼ t. salt
- 1 egg
- ½ t. vanilla
- 1¼ c. flour
- ¾ t. baking soda

Preheat oven to 375°. Combine butter and peanut butter. Add sugars, salt, egg and vanilla and beat until light and fluffy. Add dry ingredients. Shape into 1" balls and place on baking sheet. Flatten in a crisscross pattern with a fork. Bake for 9-10 minutes.

Yield: about 2 dozen

Oatmeal Cookies

- ½ c. shortening
- ½ c. sugar
- 1 egg
- 1 t. vanilla
- 1 c. oatmeal
- ¾ c. flour
- ½ t. soda
- ½ t. cinnamon
- ¼ t. salt
- ½ c. raisins or nuts (opt.)

Preheat oven to 350°. Cream shortening, sugar, eggs and vanilla. Stir in dry ingredients until blended. Add raisins or nuts if desired. Drop by tablespoons onto greased baking sheet. Bake for 10-12 minutes.

Yield: about 2 dozen

Oatmeal Chocolate Chip Cookies

- ½ c. butter
- ½ c. granulated sugar
- ½ c. brown sugar
- 1 egg
- ½ t. vanilla
- 1 ¼ c. flour
- 1 ¼ c. oatmeal
- ½ t. salt
- ½ t. soda
- 1 6-oz. package chocolate chips
- ½ c. nuts (opt.)

Preheat oven to 325°. Cream together butter and sugars. Add eggs and vanilla and beat well. Stir in dry ingredients. Add chocolate chips and nuts as desired. Drop by tablespoons onto baking sheet and bake for 8-11 minutes. Cool slightly before removing from tray.

Yield: 3 dozen

Applesauce Cookies

- ½ c. shortening
- 1 c. sugar
- 1 egg
- ½ c. applesauce
- 2 c. flour
- 1 t. soda
- ½ t. cloves
- ½ t. nutmeg
- 1 t. cinnamon
- ½ t. salt
- Raisins or chocolate chips (opt.)

Preheat oven to 400°. Cream shortening and sugar. Beat in eggs and applesauce. Stir in dry ingredients and raisins or chocolate chips if desired. Drop by tablespoons onto greased baking sheet and bake for 10-12 minutes.

Yield: 2-3 dozen

Sugar Cookies

- 1 c. sugar
- ½ c. butter
- 2 eggs
- 1/2 c. milk
- 1 t. vanilla
- ½ t. lemon extract
- ½ t. salt
- 2 t. baking powder
- 3 c. flour

Cream shortening, sugar, and eggs and beat well. Blend in milk, vanilla and lemon flavoring. Combine dry ingredients and add to batter, stirring gently to avoid over beating. Add additional flour if needed to form a very soft dough. Roll ¼" thick. Sprinkle with sugar and cut into desired shapes. Bake at 375° F. for 8-10 minutes. May also omit sugar on top and frost as desired.

Yield: 2-3 dozen cookies

Janet's Soft Sugar Cookies

- 3 c. flour
- ½ t. salt
- 2 t. baking powder
- ½ c. butter
- 1 c. sugar
- 2 eggs
- ¼ c. milk
- 2 t. vanilla
- ½ t. almond or lemon extract
- 3 T. E-Z Gel®

Preheat oven to 375°. Sift together dry ingredients and set aside.

Cream butter and sugar in large bowl with electric mixer until fluffy (10 minutes). Add eggs, milk, flavorings and E-Z Gel® and beat until light. Stir in dry ingredients to make a soft dough. Let stand for 5 minutes. Add additional flour if needed. Roll out ¼" thick and sprinkle with colored sugar (if desired). Cut into shapes. Arrange on ungreased baking sheets and bake for 8-10 minutes until edges are barely browned.

Cool for 5 minutes on baking sheet. Transfer cookies to rack and cool completely. Store in airtight container or freeze. If desired, omit sugar on top and frost.

Yield: 2-3 dozen

Snickerdoodles

- 1 c. butter, softened (for a puffier cookie use 1/2 c. shortening and 1/2 c. butter)
- 1 ½ c. sugar
- 2 eggs
- 2 t. vanilla
- 2 T. E-Z Gel®
- 2 T. water
- 2 ¾ c. flour
- 2 t. cream of tartar
- 1 t. baking soda
- ¼ t. salt

Topping:

- 2 T. sugar
- 2 t. ground cinnamon

Preheat oven to 400°. Sift together dry ingredients and set aside.

Cream together butter and sugar in large bowl with electric mixer until fluffy. Add eggs one at a time, beating after each addition. Stir in vanilla, E-Z Gel® and water. Add dry ingredients to creamed mixture, stirring until well blended. Shape into 1" balls. Mix together sugar and cinnamon. Roll dough balls in cinnamon mixture and place on an ungreased baking sheet. Bake for 8-10 minutes until lightly browned.

Cool for 5 minutes on baking sheet. Transfer cookies to rack and cool. Store in airtight container or freeze.

Yield: 3 dozen

Danish Sugar Cookies

- 1 c. sugar
- 1 c. butter
- 1 egg
- 1 t. vanilla
- 2 c. flour
- ½ t. baking soda
- ½ t. cream of tartar

Preheat oven to 325°. Cream sugar, butter, egg and vanilla until light. Add dry ingredients. Blend well. Make dough balls about the size of walnuts. Bake for about 10 minutes. These cookies also work well as a refrigerator cookies: Roll in cylinders and refrigerate or freeze. To bake, cut off ¼" slices and bake at 325° for about 10 minutes.

Yield: 2 dozen

Cakes and Icing

Cakes

Double Chocolate Cake

- 1 pkg. chocolate cake mix
- 1 (8-oz.) carton vanilla yogurt
- 1 (6-oz.) pkg. instant vanilla pudding mix
- 1 c. milk chocolate chips
- ½ c. oil
- 4 eggs
- 1 c. water

Combine all ingredients by hand in a medium mixing bowl. Spray 4-quart slow cooker with pan spray, then pour in prepared batter. Bake on high for 3-4 hours or bake on low for 6-8 hours. Serve warm with chocolate sauce and whipped cream.

Yield: 12 servings

Sponge Cake

- 5 eggs, separated
- ½ c. cold water
- 1 t. vanilla
- ¾ t. cream of tartar
- 1½ c. sugar
- 1½ c. sifted cake flour
- ½ t. baking powder
- ½ t. salt

Beat egg yolks and water with electric mixer until thick. Add sugar gradually and beat for 5 minutes. Add salt and vanilla. Beat egg whites in large glass or metal bowl until thick and foamy. Add cream of tartar and beat until stiff. Sift together dry ingredients and add to yolk mixture, then fold in beaten egg whites. Pour into UNGREASED angel food cake pan and bake for 60-70 minutes until golden brown and springs back Turn upside down to cool completely before removing from pan. Serve with fresh fruit or Seven Minute Icing.

Yield: 16 servings

Chiffon Cake

- 2¼ c. cake flour
- 1 T. baking powder
- ½ t. salt
- 1½ c. sugar
- 4 egg yolks
- ½ c. vegetable oil
- 2 t. vanilla
- ¾ c. cold water
- 6 egg whites
- ½ t. cream of tartar

Preheat oven to 325°. Sift together cake flour, baking powder, and salt. Place egg yolks in large bowl and beat until thick and lemon colored. Continue beating and incorporate 1 c. sugar, 1 T. at a time, until mixture is very thick. Pour oil in a slow stream over egg mixture and continue beating. Add vanilla. Alternately fold in dry ingredients and water with a rubber spatula. Set aside. Beat egg whites and cream of tartar in large glass or metal bowl to soft peaks. Gradually add remaining 1/3 c. sugar and beat to stiff peaks. Gently fold about 1 c. of the yolk mixture into the whites to lighten, then fold the beaten white mixture into the batter. Pour into ungreased 10" tube pan and bake for 50 minutes. Increase temperature to 350° and bake until top springs back. Immediately invert the pan onto a cake rack and cool completely in pan. Remove from pan by running a small, sharp knife around the edges and invert onto a plate. **Chocolate Chiffon Cake:** Prepare Chiffon Cake as directed, using only 2 c. flour. Add ¼ c. cocoa to sifted dry ingredients.

Yield: 16 servings

Special Chocolate Cake

- 3 egg yolks
- 1 c. sour cream
- 1 ½ c. sugar
- 2 (1-oz) squares unsweetened chocolate
- ¼ c. hot water
- 1 t. vanilla
- 1 ¾ c. cake flour
- ½ t. salt
- 1 t. baking soda
- 3 egg whites, stiffly beaten

Combine egg yolks, sour cream and sugar in large mixing bowl. Beat with electric mixer until fluffy. Melt chocolate in hot water over low heat; cool and add to first mixture with vanilla. Fold in sifted dry ingredients, then beaten egg whites. Pour into greased and floured 9" x 13" baking pan or two 9" rounds. Bake at 350° F. for 30-45 minutes.

Yield: 15 servings

German Chocolate Cake

- 1 8-oz. bar German chocolate
- ½ c. boiling water
- 1 c. margarine
- 1½ c. sugar
- 2 egg yolks
- 1 t. vanilla
- ½ t. salt
- 1 t. soda
- 2½ c. cake flour
- 1 c. sour milk
- 5 egg whites

Melt chocolate in boiling water and cool. Cream margarine, sugar, egg yolks and vanilla with electric mixer. Combine dry ingredients in small bowl. Alternately add sour milk and dry ingredients to creamed mixture. Fold in melted chocolate mixture. Whip egg whites to stiff peaks in glass or metal bowl and fold into chocolate mixture. Pour into three 8"inch greased and floured layer cake pans. Bake at 325° for 25-30 minutes. Cool in pans for 10 minutes, then turn cakes onto cooling racks. Cool for 15 minutes then frost with Coconut Pecan Frosting.

Yield: 15 servings

Texas Sheet Cake

- 2 c. flour
- 2 c. sugar
- 1 t. baking soda
- 1 c. margarine
- 1 c. water
- ¼-1/3 c. cocoa
- 2 eggs
- ½ c. buttermilk or sour milk
- 1 t. vanilla

Combine dry ingredients. Melt margarine in medium saucepan. Add cocoa and water and bring to a boil. Add to flour mixture and beat well. Add remaining ingredients and stir to combine. Pour into greased and floured 11"x17" jelly roll pan and bake at 375° for 20-25 minutes. Ice with Chocolate Fudge Frosting.

Yield: 15 servings

Jelly Roll or Torte

- 6 eggs, separated
- 1 t. vanilla
- ½ t. salt
- ½ c. sugar
- ½ c. flour
- ½ c. E-Z Gel®

Preheat oven to 325°. Prepare pans.

Jelly Roll: Spray 11"x 17" jelly roll pan with pan spray and line with waxed paper. Spray waxed paper with pan spray and sprinkle with flour.

Torte: Spray two 10-inch fluted torte pans with pan spray and sprinkle with flour.

Separate eggs, placing whites in medium glass bowl and yolks in large glass bowl. Do not allow any of the egg yolk to get into the egg whites! Add salt to egg whites and beat with electric mixer on high speed to soft peaks. Gradually add sugar and beat to stiff peaks. Add vanilla to egg yolks in large bowl and beat until light and lemon-colored. Scoop the beaten whites over the yolk mixture, spreading to the edges of the beaten yolks, then sprinkle on the flour and E-Z Gel®. Fold gently to combine.

Spread batter into pan(s) and bake for about 10-12 minutes until barely brown and springy to the touch. Cool for 5 minutes.

Jelly Roll: Turn cake out onto a kitchen towel. Remove the waxed paper and sprinkle the cake generously with powdered sugar. Place another kitchen towel on top of the cake and flip the cake right side up. Roll cake and towel together, pretty side out, and cool completely. Unroll and remove towel, then fill as desired and reroll. Refrigerate or freeze for 30 minutes or more before cutting with serrated edge knife. Jelly rolls may be filled with cheesecake filling, wrapped well in double layers of plastic wrap, and frozen for up to three months.

Torte: Remove cake from pans, using fingers as needed. Place on serving trays. Fill with and decorate with fresh fruit.

Chocolate variation: Whisk 1/3 cup cocoa powder in with flour mixture.

Yield: 18 servings

Strawberry Short Cake

Prepare jelly roll or torte as directed. Grease and flour muffin tins or use cupcake liners. Fill 2/3 full. Bake for about 8 minutes until golden brown. Cool for 5 minutes then turn out onto rack. Cool completely. Serve with fresh strawberries and whipping cream.

Angel Food Cake

- 1½ c. egg whites (about 1 dozen)
- ½ t. salt
- 1½ t. cream of tartar
- 1 t. vanilla
- ½ c. sifted sugar
- 1 c. sugar
- 1 c. sifted cake flour

Beat egg whites until foamy. Add salt, cream of tartar and vanilla and beat until soft peaks are formed. Gradually add ½ c. sifted sugar and beat to stiff, but not dry peaks. Sift together 1 c. sugar and 1 c. sifted cake flour three times. Gently fold in sugar/flour mixture, stirring just until well blended.

Turn batter in an UNGREASED 10" tube pan. Cut through batter to remove air pockets. Bake in preheated 350° F oven for 35-45 minutes until golden brown–crust will not feel sticky. Invert to cool.

Yield: 16 servings

Chocolate Flake Angel Food Cake: Prepare Angel Food Cake as directed, folding in ½ c. grated chocolate during few seconds of folding.

Orange Angel Food Cake: Prepare Angel Food Cake as directed, substituting 1 T. orange juice for vanilla. Add ½ t. grated zest of orange during last few seconds of folding.

Peppermint Angel Food Cake: Prepare Angel Food Cake as directed, adding _ c. crushed peppermint candy during last few seconds of folding.

Lemon-Coconut Angel Food Cake: Prepare Angel Food Cake as directed, adding ½ c. shredded coconut and ½ t. grated lemon zest during last few seconds of folding.

Chocolate Angel Food Cake: Prepare Angel Food Cake as directing, sifting ¼ c. cocoa into sugar/flour mixture.

Almond Angel Food Cake: Prepare Angel Food Cake as directed, substituting ½ t. almond extract for ½ t. vanilla.

Pumpkin Cake

Crust:

- 1 white or yellow cake mix (reserve 1 cup)
- 1 egg
- ½ c. melted butter

Filling:

- 1 (29 oz.) can 100% pure pumpkin
- 1 ½ c. sugar
- 1 t. salt
- 2 t. ground cinnamon
- 1 t. ground ginger
- ½ t. ground cloves
- 4 large eggs
- 1 (12 oz) can evaporated milk

Topping:

- 1 c. reserved cake mix
- 2 T. sugar
- 1 t. cinnamon
- 1/4 c. softened butter

Preheat oven to 350°. Mix together the crust ingredients and press mixture on the bottom of a 9x13 inch cake pan.

Combine pumpkin, sugar, salt, and spices in a large bowl. Mix to combine. Add eggs and mix for an additional minute until incorporated. Gradually mix in evaporated milk. Pour pumpkin mixture over unbaked crust. Combine topping ingredients together in a small bowl. Mix until crumbly. Sprinkle topping over pumpkin mixture.

Bake for 1 hour until the pumpkin cake is set and tests done in the center. Allow to cool and serve with sweetened whipped cream.

Yield: 16-20 servings

White Wedding Cake

- 1 ½ c. butter
- 4 c. sugar
- 8 eggs, separated
- 4 t. vanilla
- 7 c. cake flour
- 2 T. baking powder
- 2 t. salt
- 3 ½ c. milk

Preheat the oven to 325 F. Grease and flour one 16 x 2 inch round cake pan.

Cream together the butter and sugar until well blended. Add egg yolks, one at a time, and beat well. Add vanilla. Continuing beating in stand mixer for at least 10 minutes until mixture becomes creamy and pale yellow. Sift together dry ingredients. Add dry ingredients and milk alternatively to creamed mixture. In a separate bowl, whip egg white to stiff, but not dry, peaks. Gently fold into cake mixture until full incorporated. Pour batter into prepared cake pan and bake for about 1 hour until cake tests done. Turn off oven and set time for 10 minutes. Remove cake from oven and let cool for 15 minutes, then remove from pan.

Yield: 1 16 inch round cake, approximately 20 servings

Lemon Wedding Cake

Prepare White Wedding Cake as instructed but add 2 t. lemon extract to batter with vanilla and top with lemon frosting.

Carrot Cake

- 3 eggs
- 1 ¼ c. oil
- 2 c. sugar
- 2 c. grated carrots
- 1 15-oz. can crushed pineapple (undrained)
- 3 c. flour
- 1½ t. baking soda
- ½ t. salt
- 1 t. cinnamon
- 1 ½ c. nuts
- 1 t. vanilla

Preheat oven to 350°. Cream together eggs, oil and sugar. Add carrots and pineapple. Add dry ingredients, nuts and vanilla. Pour into greased and floured 9" x 13" cake pan or two 9" round cake pans. Bake sheet cake for 1 hour, round for 45-50 minutes. Frost with Cream Cheese Frosting.

Yield: 15 servings

Banana Cake

- 2/3 c. butter
- 1 1/3 c. sugar
- 2 eggs
- 2½ c. cake flour
- 1¼ t. baking powder
- 1 t. soda
- 1 t. salt
- 1¼ c. mashed bananas
- 2/3 c. buttermilk

Beat together shortening, sugar and eggs until light and fluffy. Add sifted dry ingredients alternately with mixture of buttermilk and bananas. Fold in chopped walnuts if desired. Turn into greased and floured 9" x 13" baking pan and bake at 350° for about 30 minutes until cake tests done. Frost with Cream Cheese Icing if desired.

Yield: 15 servings

Microwave Gingerbread Cake

- ¼ c. butter
- 1 T. sugar
- 1 egg
- ½ c. molasses
- ½ c. boiling water
- 1 ¼ c. flour
- 1 t. cinnamon
- ½ t. baking soda
- ½ t. ginger
- ¼ t. salt

Cream butter and sugar with electric mixer. Add egg and molasses and beat well. Stir in boiling water. Combine flour, cinnamon, baking soda, ginger, and salt. Stir flour mixture into creamed mixture. Pour into a greased 9 inch microwave safe pie plate. Microwave on HIGH heat about 7-8 minutes, or until a toothpick inserted in center comes out clean. To cook evenly use a microwave with a turn table or rotate the cake every few minutes. Cover with wax paper and let stand for 5 minutes. Invert onto a plate and serve with warm lemon sauce or powdered sugar glaze.

Yield: 6-8 servings

Icing, Frosting, and Filling

Seven Minute Icing

Combine 1 c. sugar, 2 T. white corn syrup and 1/3 c. water in medium saucepan. Bring to a boil and cook for exactly 3 minutes. Meanwhile beat 2 egg whites in large bowl to form soft peaks. Gradually add hot sugar mixture to egg whites, beating constantly with electric mixer. Continue beating until soft peaks form and icing will spread well. Beat in ½ t. vanilla or flavoring as desired.

Yield: Icing for one angel food cake, one 9" x 13" cake or two 9" round layers.

Cream Cheese Frosting

- 3 oz. softened cream cheese
- 2 T. butter
- ½ lb powdered sugar
- ¼ c. milk (approx.)

Beat cream cheese and butter with electric mixer until smooth. Add powdered sugar, and 2 T. milk, beating well. Stir in additional milk 1 T. at a time for desired consistency.

Yield: frosting for 1 single layer 9" cake or 12 cupcakes

Lemon Butter Frosting

- 1/3 c. butter, softened
- 3 c. powdered sugar
- ½ teaspoon grated lemon peel
- About 2 tablespoons lemon juice

Mix butter and powdered sugar. Beat in lemon peel and lemon juice until of spreading consistency.

Yield: Frosting for one 13x9 inch or two 9 inch round cakes.

Coconut Pecan Frosting

Combine 1 c. sugar, 3 egg yolks, 2 c. evaporated milk and ½ c. butter in medium saucepan. Cook and stir over low heat until thick, 10-12 minutes. Remove from heat and add 1 c. coconut, 1 c. chopped pecans and 1 t. vanilla. Stir well to combine.

Yield: Frosting for two 9-inch cakes

Chocolate Fudge Frosting

Combine ½ c. butter, ¼ c. milk, and 3 T. cocoa in small saucepan. Bring to a boil. Remove from heat and add 1 lb. powdered sugar and 1 t. vanilla. Beat well. Add additional powdered sugar if necessary to make a creamy frosting.

Yield: Frosting for two 9-inch cakes

Chocolate-Almond Filling

Beat 1 c. chilled whipping cream, ¼ c. powdered sugar and 2 T. cocoa in chilled bowl until stiff. Beat in ½ t. vanilla. Fold in ¼ c. toasted sliced almonds. Spread baked cake roll with whipped cream mixture. Roll up; frost if desired.

Yield: Filling for one jelly roll.

Candies and Confections

Divinity

- 2 c. sugar
- 1/2 c. light corn syrup
- 1/2 c. water
- 2 egg whites
- 1 t. vanilla
- 1 c. walnuts (opt)

Line a 15" x 10" jellyroll pan with waxed paper; set aside.

In a heavy saucepan heat sugar, corn syrup, and water until it will spin a thread. While heating the sugar mixture beat egg whites with a pinch of salt. Pour hot sugar slowly into beaten egg white with mixer running. If needed put mixture back on stove for a few seconds after each addition. Add vanilla and when almost set, add nuts. Scoop by teaspoons onto waxed paper.

Yield: about 40 pieces

Divinity Eggs

Prepare divinity as directed. Scrape divinity onto waxed paper and let stand until set. Using buttered hands, gently press divinity into buttered egg mold, *or* butter hands and form divinity into egg shapes. Remove from mold and transfer to waxed paper-lined tray. Dip into tempered dipping chocolate.

English Toffee

- 1 lb. sweet cream butter
- 2 ½ c. sugar
- ½ c. water
- ¼ c. light corn syrup
- 1 c. chopped almonds

Butter a 12" x 18" baking sheet; set aside. Combine butter, sugar, water and corn syrup in heavy 3-quart saucepan. Place over high heat and stir with a wooden spoon until butter melts and mixture comes to a rolling boil. Reduce heat to low and cook to a soft-crack stage (295° F). Stir in chopped almonds and pour onto greased baking sheet. Spread to uniform thickness while hot.

When toffee is firm, sprinkle with ½ bag milk chocolate chips or grated chocolate; spread when melted and top with chopped nuts. Break into pieces to serve.

Yield: about 70 pieces

Cathedral Window Candy

- 1 (12-oz.) pkg. semi-sweet chocolate chips
- ½ c. butter or margarine
- 2 eggs
- 1 (10-oz.) pkg. colored miniature marshmallows
- 1 c. coarsely chopped nuts
- crushed graham crackers, coconut, powdered sugar, ground nuts, etc.

Melt chocolate chips and butter together over low heat in medium saucepan. Remove from heat and beat in eggs. Return to heat and cook for 1 minute. Let stand to cool for 5 minutes. Pour chocolate mixture over marshmallows and nuts, stirring to coat well.

Spread out 4 sheets of waxed paper 18 inches long and sprinkle with crushed graham crackers, coconut, nuts, or powdered sugar as desired. Spoon marshmallow mixture onto crumbs in a log shape about 2" in diameter. Roll log in crumbs to coat and wrap with waxed paper, sealing well. Repeat with remaining mixture and waxed paper to form four logs.

Freeze for at least 30 minutes. Cut into ¾" slices to serve.

Yield: About 80 pieces

Cream Fondant

- 1 c. whipping cream
- ½ c. milk
- ½ c. light corn syrup
- 4½ c. sugar
- ¼ t. salt

Combine ingredients in order listed in heavy saucepan. Place over high heat and stir until mixture boils. Wash down crystals and cook to soft ball (232°). Pour onto marble slab and cool to lukewarm. Work with spatula until candy creams. Knead with hands until smooth, adding coloring and flavoring as desired. Form into ball and store in tightly covered container overnight. Roll into centers and dip with tempered dipping chocolate.

Yield: 120 pieces

Water Fondant

- 4 c. sugar
- 1/3 c. light corn syrup
- ¼ t. cream of tartar
- ¼ c. butter
- 1/8 t. salt
- 1 1/3 c. water

Follow directions for Cream Fondant, cooking to a firm soft ball (234°). Add 1 c. marshmallow cream to lukewarm candy mixture and work until candy creams. Color and flavor as desired. Store in tightly covered container. Roll into centers and dip with tempered dipping chocolate.

Yield: 120 pieces

Opera Creams

- 2 c. sugar
- 2/3 c. heavy cream
- ¼ c. white corn syrup
- ¼ t. salt

Combine ingredients in heavy saucepan. Bring to a gentle boil, stirring constantly. Cook to a soft ball (232° F). Remove from heat and cool to lukewarm without stirring. Beat with a wooden spoon until mixture loses gloss; add flavorings and nuts as desired and spread into buttered baking pan to cool. Cut into squares and dip if desired.

Yield: about 50 pieces

Peanut Butter Bon Bons

Combine 1 c. peanut butter, ¼ c. soft butter, and 2 c. powdered sugar to make a dough-like consistency. Roll into small balls and set aside. Temper 1½ lbs. dipping chocolate. Dip peanut butter balls in tempered chocolate and let cool until set.

Favorite Caramels

- 1 c. granulated sugar
- 1 c. brown sugar
- ½ t. salt
- 1 c. light corn syrup
- 1 c. whipping cream
- 1/4 c. E-Z Gel®
- 1 c. whipping cream
- 1 c. granulated sugar
- 2 t. vanilla

Combine 1 cup granulated sugar and brown sugar, salt, corn syrup and 1 c. cream in a heavy sauce pan. (At least 4 quart capacity.) Bring to a boil over medium high heat, stirring constantly. Gradually add E-Z Gel®, using a whisk to mix it in fully. Cook at a gentle boil for 6 minutes until mixture thickens, then add remaining 1 c. whipping cream and 1 c. granulated sugar. Cook to desired firmness.

For caramel sauce: boil for 8 minutes, stir in vanilla. Store, covered, in refrigerator for up to two weeks.

For caramel coating boil for 10 minutes. Stir in vanilla. Store, covered, in refrigerator for up to weeks. Reheat in microwave as needed.

For wonderful caramel popcorn or popcorn balls, boil for 12 minutes. Stir in vanilla and your choice of nuts. Pour over 6 quarts popped popcorn, stirring to coat. For extra gooey popcorn balls, add 4 c. miniature marshmallows to the popped popcorn before adding caramel mixture. For popcorn pieces spread onto lightly oiled baking sheets and let cool. For popcorn balls, shape while warm. Let cool, then wrap in cellophane or plastic wrap.

Yield: about 50 pieces

Mom's Caramels

- 1 c. light corn syrup
- 2 c. sugar
- 3 c. whipping cream (divided into thirds)
- ¼ t. salt
- 1 t. vanilla, if desired
- 1 c. chopped pecans

Combine corn syrup, sugar, 1 cup cream, and salt in heavy 4-quart saucepan. Cook over low heat to medium hard ball (228° F). Gradually add second cup cream and cook to medium hard ball (228° F). Add remaining cream and cook to medium hard ball (228° F). Remove from heat and stir in vanilla and nuts, if desired. Pour into a buttered 9" x 13" cake pan and cool until firm.

Yield: about 60 pieces

Microwave Caramels

- 1 c. butter, melted
- 1 (14 oz.) can sweetened condensed milk
- 1 c. light corn syrup
- 1 (1 lb.) pkg. light brown sugar
- 1 t. vanilla

Melt butter in large microwave safe, heat-resistant glass bowl. Stir in sweetened condensed milk, light corn syrup, and brown sugar. Microwave on HIGH for 15 minutes, stirring every three minutes. Continue cooking, checking every 1 minute, until candy reaches hard ball stage. Pour into lightly buttered 9x13 inch pan and refrigerate until set.

Yield: about 24 pieces

Chocolate Truffles

- 1 ½ pounds (about 4 ½ c.) milk chocolate, melted (110° F/45°C)
- 1 cup whipping cream
- 1 ½ teaspoons vanilla

Line an 8-inch square baking pan with plastic wrap; set aside. Place melted chocolate in a medium-size bowl. In a 1-quart saucepan, scald cream. Remove from heat and let cool for 5 minutes. Stir in vanilla. Beat chocolate with an electric mixer. Stop mixer and pour cream all at once over chocolate. Continue beating, cleaning sides and bottom of bowl several times with rubber scraper, until mixture is smooth and well-blended; this takes no more than 1 to 2 minutes. Pour into prepared pan and refrigerate 6 hours or until firm. Cut into 1-inch squares and serve immediately. Store in refrigerator.

These make great centers for a dipped chocolate, or pieces can be rolled in sugar, nuts, coconut or other fun additions.

Yield: 64 pieces

Mint Truffles: Prepare Chocolate Truffles as directed adding 5 drops oil of peppermint in place of vanilla. Dip in tempered dipping chocolate.

Yield: 64 pieces

Chocolate Fudge

- 2 c. sugar
- 2/3 c. evaporated milk
- 2 oz. unsweetened baking chocolate
- dash salt
- 1 T. light corn syrup
- 2 T. butter
- 1 t. vanilla

Butter sides of heavy 4-quart saucepan. Combine sugar, evaporated milk, chocolate, salt and corn syrup. Cook over medium heat, stirring constantly until chocolate is melted and sugar is dissolved. Cook to soft ball stage (236° F), stirring only to prevent scorching. Remove from heat and add butter, but don't stir. Cool to lukewarm on a wire rack. DO NOT STIR!!!

When mixture is cool, beat vigorously with a wooden spoon until fudge stiffens and loses its gloss. Push from saucepan (do not scrape sides) into a buttered baking pan.

Yield: about 40 pieces

Easy Chocolate Fudge

- 1 (12-ounce) package chocolate chips (semi-sweet)
- 1 (7-ounce) jar marshmallow creme
- 1 (12-ounce) can evaporated milk
- ½ c. butter or margarine
- 4 c. sugar
- ½ t. salt
- 1 T. E-Z Gel®

Butter a 9" x 13" baking pan; set aside. Combine chocolate pieces and marshmallow cream in a large bowl; set aside. In a heavy 4-quart saucepan, combine sugar, salt, and E-Z Gel® until well combined. Add evaporated milk and butter. Place over medium heat and stir occasionally with a wooden spoon until mixture comes to a boil. Boil, stirring occasionally, for 7 minutes (soft ball).

Pour over chocolate-marshmallow creme mixture. Using a wooden spoon, beat until mixture is creamy. Stir in nuts if desired. Pour fudge into prepared pan. Refrigerate 6 hours or until firm. Cut into 1-inch squares. Keeps well for several weeks in the refrigerator.

Yield: about 120 pieces

Rocky Road Fudge

Prepare Easy Chocolate Fudge as directed. Add 2 c. miniature marshmallows with nuts.

White Fudge

- 6 c. sugar
- 2 c. cream
- 1 c. milk
- ½ c. light corn syrup
- 1/4 t. salt
- 1 c. butter
- 2 t. vanilla

Line a 9 x 13 inch baking pan with waxed paper. Butter well and set aside. Combine sugar, cream, milk, corn syrup, and salt in a heavy, six quart Dutch oven. Stir to combine. Bring to a boil over high heat. Reduce heat to medium high and cook to a firm ball. Pour into the bowl of a 5-quart stand mixer and add butter and vanilla. Beat well until mixture cools and begins to lose its gloss. Add nuts, if desired, and pour into prepared pan, smoothing the surface as necessary. Allow to stand for 4-6 hours to harden.

Yield: about 60 pieces

Peanut Brittle

- 1 ½ c. sugar
- ½ c. light corn syrup
- ½ c. water
- 1 c. peanuts
- 1 T. butter
- ½ t. vanilla
- 1 ½ t. baking soda

Butter a 15" x 10" jellyroll pan or 15-inch pizza pan; set aside. In a heavy 3-quart saucepan, combine corn syrup, water and sugar. Place over high heat and stir with a wooden spoon until mixture comes to a boil. When syrup starts to thicken, stir in peanuts. Stirring constantly, cook until the peanuts smell cooked and the syrup bubbles are a pale straw color.

Remove from heat and stir in butter and vanilla. *Use caution as this will cause steam and could burn your hand.* Stir in baking soda until it foams. Pour onto baking sheet and allow to cool for several minutes.

Using 2 forks, or buttered finger tips, begin stretching the edges away from the mass of brittle. Work your way around the pan, pulling off pieces as you stretch. Place these pieces upside down as this will cause the peanuts to stay in the center of the candy, rather than sink to the bottom. Continue in this manner until all the brittle has been stretched. Allow to cool completely. Store in airtight containers.

Yield: 1 pound

Candy Canes

- 6 c. sugar
- 3 c. cold water
- 2 T. light corn syrup
- 1/8 t. salt
- 1 t. cream of tartar

Combine sugar, water, corn syrup and salt in heavy saucepan. Heat to a boil, stirring constantly until sugar is dissolved then remove spoon from pan and bring to a rolling boil. Wash down the crystals, then add the cream of tartar. Boil to a hard crack stage. Pour most of the sugar mixture onto a greased baking sheet or marble slab and the rest into a buttered pie plate. DO NOT SCRAPE THE PAN OR DISTURB THE MIXTURE UNTIL ALMOST COOL!!!

Turn in the edges and add flavoring as desired. (Approx. 12 drops flavored oil in larger portion and 6 drops in smaller amount). Add food coloring as desired to mixture in pie plate. Gather the candy from the baking pan into a ball and pull until creamy, then shape into a ball. Meanwhile mix the flavor and color into the mixture in the pie plate and shape it into a rope. Wrap the colored stripe around the creamy ball and pull them together, twisting to form the traditional stripe.

Roll smooth on a wooden board and cut into desired lengths. A little cornstarch may keep the candy from sticking to hands or board. If the sticks get too cool to work with before they are shaped, heat on a wooden cutting board in a warm oven to soften. Store in tightly sealed container!!!!!

Yield: Lots!!!

Butter Mints

- 1 c. boiling water
- 3 c. sugar
- ½ c. butter (no substitutions)
- 5 drops oil of peppermint
- 3 drops food coloring (opt.)

Combine boiling water and sugar in a heavy 4-quart saucepan and bring to a boil. Cover with tight fitting lid and continue boiling for 3 minutes. Uncover and wash down the crystals on the sides of the pan and the spoon. Add thermometer and cook to soft ball stage (240° F). Add butter and cook to firm ball (254° F).

Remove from heat and pour onto buttered marble slab to cool. Drop peppermint oil and food coloring onto hot candy, then fold cooled edges into the hot center. Repeat until the candy can be gathered into a ball, incorporating the peppermint oil and food coloring. Stretch like taffy until the candy is hard to pull and loses its gloss. Twist into long rope-like strands and cut into square pillows with scissors or kitchen shears.

Sprinkle lightly with powdered sugar if necessary to prevent sticking. Place in tightly sealed container and set aside for two or three days to become smooth and creamy.

Yield: about 120 pieces

Old-Fashioned Taffy

- 2 c. sugar
- ½ c. light corn syrup
- ½ t. cream of tartar
- 2/3 c. water
- 1/8 t. salt
- 5 drops flavored oil
- food color (optional)

Combine first five ingredients in heavy 3-quart saucepan and bring to a boil over high heat. Wash down crystal with hot water and pastry brush. Boil to firm ball (265° F). Pour onto buttered cookie sheet. When cool enough to handle, add flavoring and color and put until light and creamy. Stretch out, cut, and wrap in waxed paper squares. Store in an airtight container.

Yield: about 40 pieces

Pies and Puddings

Basic Pie Crust

- 2 c. all-purpose OR pastry flour
- ½ t. salt
- 1 c. shortening or butter, or half of each depending on desired tenderness and flavor
- Ice water to make soft dough

Combine flour and salt. Cut in shortening to the size of peas. Gradually add just enough ice water to form a soft dough. Divide into two disks, wrap in plastic wrap and refrigerate for 10 minutes. Shape as desired on lightly floured waxed paper or silicon sheet. Bake single crust pie shells as directed at 400° F. Bake double crust pie according to filling instructions.

It's important to work with cold shortening and cold tools when making flakey pie crust.

Yield: 2 single-crust pie shells or 1 double-crust pie

Tart Shells

- 1 c. all-purpose flour
- ¼ t. salt
- 2 T. sugar (opt.)
- ½ c. cold butter, cut into ½″ cubes
- 1 egg, slightly beaten
- ¼ c. milk

Combine flour and salt in medium bowl. Cut in butter until evenly distributed. Combine egg and milk in small bowl. Add gradually to flour mixture, tossing lightly with a fork to distribute. Form into a ball, cover with plastic wrap and refrigerate for 30 minutes or freeze for 10 minutes. Divide into walnut-size balls and press into 2″ tart pans, pricking well. Freeze for 10 minutes. Preheat oven to 425° and bake for about 10 minutes until light brown. Let cool for 10 minutes and remove from tart pans to cool completely. Fill as desired.

Yield: 20 small tart shells

No Fail Pie Crust

- 5 c. all-purpose flour
- 1 t. salt
- 2 c. shortening
- 1 egg
- 1 T. vinegar plus ice water to equal 1 cup

Combine flour and salt in large bowl. Cut in shortening until mixture is crumbly with lumps the size of peas. Combine egg and water-vinegar mixture. Gradually add to flour mixture, adding just enough to form a workable dough. Divide dough into six balls and flatten slightly, taking care not to overwork. Wrap each flattened disk in plastic wrap and refrigerate for 10 minutes. Remove one disk from refrigerator at a time and roll between floured squares of waxed paper or on lightly floured board to ¼" thickness and diameter about 1" larger than pie pan.

To bake blind (single crust, no filling), preheat oven to 425° F. Fold dough in quarters and transfer to pie pan. Trim and finish edge as desired and prick entire surface with tines of fork. Refrigerate for 10 minutes. Method 1: Remove from refrigerator and line prepared crust with waxed paper. Fill about half way with pie weights, dried beans, rice, etc. Bake for about 10 minutes then remove waxed paper and weights and cook an additional 5 minutes or until golden brown. If necessary, shield the edges with foil if they are browning too fast. Method 2: Remove from refrigerator and bake for 10-12 minutes. If the crust begins to bubble in the oven, prick lightly to release. Cool completely before adding desired filling. Yield: 12 single crust pie shells.

To bake a double crust pie, preheat oven to 350° F. Fold one crust in quarters and transfer to pie pan. Refrigerate bottom crust while preparing filling and top crust. Prepare filling as desired. Roll top crust in same manner as bottom crust. Fold into fourths and cut slits to vent. Remove bottom crust from refrigerator and fill with prepared filling. Transfer prepared top crust onto filling and trim edges about ¾" larger than pie pan. (Opt: Brush bottom edge lightly with milk to guarantee seal.) Fold top edges under edges of bottom crust and finish edge as desired. Bake as directed for desired filling.

Yield: 3 double-crust pies

Meringue Shells

- 3 large egg whites (room temperature)
- ½ t. cream of tartar
- ¾ c. sugar
- 2 t. vanilla

Preheat oven to 275° F. Beat egg whites to soft peaks in a glass or metal bowl. Add cream of tartar and ¼ c. sugar and beat for 1 minutes. Gradually add the remaining sugar and beat to stiff, but not dry peaks. Fold in vanilla. Drop by rounded spoonfuls onto a parchment-lined baking sheet (about 1 t. for bite-size treats, 1 T. for dessert servings), forming round nests. Bake for about 15 minutes, then reduce heat to 250° and bake an additional 20-30 minutes until dry. If time allows, turn oven off and allow shells to cool completely.

Fill with whipped cream, ice cream, or pudding. Top with fresh fruit or chocolate glaze if desired. Serve immediately.

Yield: 12 medium shells

Cream Puffs

This is a versatile recipe, but it does not work well when doubled!

- ¾ c. water
- ½ c. butter or margarine
- ½ t. salt
- 1 c. flour
- 4 large eggs OR 5 medium eggs

Preheat oven to 375°. Combine water, butter and salt in a medium saucepan. Bring to a boil, then add the flour all at once, stirring constantly to make a stiff dough. Remove from heat and stir to cool for 1 minute. Add eggs one at a time, beating well after each addition. Stir until mixture is smooth and creamy.

Drop by spoonfuls onto greased or parchment-lined baking sheet (about 1 teaspoon for appetizers, 1 tablespoon for individual servings). Bake in oven until golden brown and dry (small: 25-30 minutes; large: 35-40 minutes). If time allows, turn oven off and leave cream puffs in oven for 1 hour.

Fill with sweetened whipped cream, pudding, or desired filling. Drizzle with chocolate glaze or sprinkle with powdered sugar if desired.

Yield: 30 appetizer puffs or 12 individual puffs

Chocolate Glaze: Combine 1 cup semi-sweet chocolate chips and 2 tablespoons butter or margarine. Melt on high in microwave oven, stopping to stir every ten seconds until smooth. Do not overheat. Gradually stir in ¼ cup whipping cream. Cool slightly, then drizzle over filled cream puffs.

Cream Cheese Filling: Combine 3 oz. cream cheese (room temperature), ½ c. powdered sugar, and ½ t. vanilla in medium bowl. Beat until smooth and creamy. Gradually add 1 c. whipping cream and beat to stiff peaks.

Yield: 2 cups

Lemon Glaze: Combine the juice of one lemon (2 tablespoons), ½ cup sugar, and 1 cup water in small bowl. Gradually add 4 tablespoons E-Z Gel®, stirring constantly with wire whisk. Refrigerate for 5 minutes to thicken.

Yield: About 1 cup

Five Minute Fresh Strawberry Pie

- 1 c. sugar
- 1 pkg. unsweetened strawberry Koolaid
- 2 c. cold water
- 10-12 T. E-Z Gel®
- 5-6 c. stemmed, sliced strawberries
- 2 baked 9" pie shell

Add sugar and drink mix to water in medium bowl and stir until dissolved. Gradually add E-Z Gel®, stirring constantly with a wire whisk. Add 1 t. lemon juice if desired. Fold in strawberries and turn into baked pie shells. Chill until set. Garnish with whipped cream and a strawberry fan. Refrigerate until ready to serve.

Yield: Two 9" pies

Cherry Dump Cobbler

- 1 can cherry or apple pie filling
- 1 (20 oz) can crushed pineapple (not drained)
- 1 pkg. white cake mix
- 3/4 cup butter, melted

Butter a 9x13 inch baking pan. Spread pie filling in pan. Spread pineapple and liquid plus 2 T. water over cherries. Sprinkle dry cake mix over pineapple. Drizzle the melted butter over the cake mix. Bake for 20 minutes at 350° until golden brown.

Easy Fresh Peach Pie

- 5 c. peeled, sliced ripe peaches
- 2/3 c. sugar
- 1/4 c. lemon juice
- 1/2 t. ground nutmeg
- 1/4 c. E-Z Gel®
- 1 baked 9" pie crust

Sprinkle ripe peaches with sugar, lemon juice, and nutmeg. Cover with plastic wrap or lid and let stand for 30 minutes. Drain peach juice into small bowl and gradually add E-Z Gel®, stirring until smooth and shiny. Gently fold in peaches. Turn into baked pie crust adn refrigerate until ready to serve. Garnish with whipped cream.

Yield: 1 9" pie

Oven Baked Peach Pie

- 5 c. peeled, sliced fresh peaches
- 1/4 c. lemon juice
- 2/3 c. sugar mixed with 3 T. ThickGel®
- 2 unbaked 9" pie crust

Preheat oven to 400°. Sprinkle peach slices with lemon juice. Combine sugar and ThickGel® in small bowl, then gradually add to peaches, stirring gently. Turn into unbaked pastry shell. Cover with top crust and seal edges. Vent and decorate as desired. Brush with milk or egg wash, and sprinkle with sugar. Bake for 40 minutes until crust is golden brown.

Easy Apple Pie

- 6 c. peeled, sliced cooking apples
- 2/3 c. sugar mixed with 1/3 c. E-Z Gel®
- 1 t. cinnamon
- 1 pkg. (to make 1 c.) spiced cider mix
- 1 c. water
- 1 baked 9" pie shell

Peel, core and slice apples into microwave safe bowl. Cover loosely and microwave on high for 10 minutes, stirring once. Combine sugar, cinnamon, and cider mix. Add water and stir until sugar is dissolved. Gradually add E-Z Gel® , stirring constantly with wire whisk. Fold thickened mixture into blanched apple slices. Turn into baked pie shell and refrigerate. Garnish with whipped cream.

Yield: One 9" pie

Fresh Apple Pie

- 3½ c. blanched, fresh apples in ¼" slices
- ¾ c. sugar
- ½ t. cinnamon
- 1/8 t. nutmeg (opt.)
- 3 T. cornstarch OR 3 T. ThickGel® OR
- 6 T. flour
- ½ c. cold water
- ½ c. apple juice
- 2 T. bottled lemon juice
- dough for one double crust pie

Peel, core and slice apples into medium bowl. Cover with plastic wrap and microwave on high for 5 minutes. Shake bowl to stir apple slices and microwave until apples are tender. Combine dry ingredients in medium saucepan. Add water, apple juice, and lemon juice and cook on medium heat until thick and bubbly. Fold in drained apple slices. Turn into unbaked pie crust. Cover with top crust and seal edges well. Prick and decorate as desired. Brush lightly with milk, avoiding crimped edges, and sprinkle lightly with coarse sugar. Bake at 400° F for 20 minutes, reduce heat to 350° F and bake 30-40 minutes until crust in golden brown.

Yield: One double crust pie

Apple Crisp for One

Filling:

- 1 medium cooking apple
- 2-3 drops lemon juice
- 1 T. sugar
- ¼ t. ground cinnamon

Crumb Topping:

- 2 T. flour
- 2 T. rolled oats
- 2 T. brown sugar
- 1 T. softened butter

Peel and core apple and cut into uniform ¼" slices. Place in 4" round casserole dish. Sprinkle with lemon juice. Combine sugar and cinnamon. Add to apples and toss to coat. Combine dry ingredients for crumb topping. Cut in butter with fork until the mixture is crumbly.

Method One: Cover prepared filling (no topping) loosely with plastic wrap and microwave on high for 2 minutes. Stir gently, then sprinkle with crumb topping mixture and bake uncovered in preheated oven at 375° for 15-20 minutes until apples are tender and topping is crispy.

Method Two: Sprinkle crumb topping over apple/cinnamon sugar mixture and bake uncovered in preheated oven at 375° for 30-40 minutes until apples are tender and topping is crispy.

Yield: 1 serving

Apple Crisp for Six to Eight

Follow directions above for filling using 6 medium cooking apples, 1 T. lemon juice, ¼ c. sugar, and 1 t. cinnamon. Place mixture in 8" square casserole dish. Make the crumb topping as directed using ¾ c. flour, 1 c. rolled oats, 1 c. brown sugar, 1 t. cinnamon, and ½ c. softened butter or margarine. Sprinkle topping over filling and bake uncovered at 375° for 40-45 minutes until apples are tender and topping is crispy.

Yield: 6-8 servings

Baked Apple Pudding

- 2 c. sugar
- 1 c. butter
- 2 eggs
- 2 c. flour
- 2 t. soda
- 1 t. cinnamon and ½ t. nutmeg
- 1 t. salt
- 6 large cooking apples, peeled and grated
- ½ -1 c. chopped nuts

Cream together sugar, margarine and eggs with electric mixer until sugar is dissolved and mixture is light. Combine dry ingredients and add to creamed mixture. Fold in grated apple and nuts. Pour in a greased 9" x 13" cake pan and bake at 375° for 50-60 minutes until cake tests done. Serve with ice cream and warm lemon, vanilla, or caramel sauce.

Yield: 6-8 servings

Apple Pie Bars

- 6 c. flour
- ½ t. baking powder
- 2 t. salt
- 1 c. cold butter, cut into ½″ cubes
- 1 c. shortening
- about ¾ c. + 2 T. ice water
- 2 quarts apple pie filling

Combine flour, baking powder and salt. Add butter and shortening and cut into dry ingredients to the consistency of coarse meal. Add ¾ c. ice water and toss gently until the water is evenly incorporated. If too dry, add additional 2 T. ice water. Turn out onto a floured board. Knead dough just enough to make it cling together and cut into two pieces. Roll one piece large enough to form the bottom of a 11″ x 17″ jelly roll pan. Transfer dough to baking pan and trim sides. Prepare top crust as bottom crust. Fill bottom crust with 2 quarts prepared apple pie filling, add top crust and crimp. Whip 2 egg whites to a froth and brush pastry surface. Vent top crust by making decorative holes with a sharp knife. Bake at 400° F for 15 minutes or until top is browned, then turn oven down to 350° and bake another 30 minutes. Remove from oven. Let cool 15 minutes while preparing a powdered sugar glaze. Drizzle glaze over pie bars. Let cool.

Yield: 24 servings

Cherry Pie Filling

- 3 1/3 c. fresh or frozen sour cherries
- 1 c. sugar
- ¼ c. + 1 T. ThickGel® OR cornstarch
- 1 1/3 c. water or juice from cherries
- ¼ t. almond extract (opt.)
- 1 T. + 1 t. lemon juice

Rinse and pit fresh cherries or thaw frozen cherries. Combine sugar and ThickGel® in large kettle with water or juice from cherries. If desired, add almond extract. Stir mixture and cook over medium heat until mixture thickens and begins to bubble. Add lemon juice and boil 1 minute, stirring constantly. Fold in cherries. Cool before filling prepared pie crust.

This filling is also excellent in black forest cake, or warmed and poured over ice cream.

Yield: Filling for one double crust pie

Pecan Pie

- 1 c. sugar
- 2 T. flour or 1 T. Flour and ThickGel®
- 2 eggs
- 2 T. butter, melted
- dash of salt
- 1 c. light corn syrup
- 1 c. broken pecans
- 1 c. whole pecan halves
- 1 t. vanilla
- 1 unbaked 9" pie shell

Preheat oven to 400° F. Add sugar and flour to eggs and beat well. Add butter, vanilla, salt and corn syrup. Add broken pecans and turn into unbaked pie shell. Arrange whole pecans on top. Bake for 15 minutes at 400° F then reduce heat to 350° F and bake an additional 60-70 minutes.

Yield: 1 9-inch pie

Lemon Meringue Pie

- 1 1/3 c. sugar
- 6 T. cornstarch
- dash salt
- 1 ¼ c. water
- 3 egg yolks, slightly beaten
- 1/3 c. lemon juice
- 2 T. butter or margarine
- 2 t. finely grated lemon zest
- 1 9-inch baked pie shell
- 3 egg whites
- ½ c. sugar
- ½ t. cream of tartar

Combine sugar, cornstarch, salt and water in heavy saucepan and bring to a boil, stirring constantly. Cook until thickened. Stir about ½ c. cooked mixture into egg yolks, then stir egg yolks into filling. Cook for 3 minutes, stirring constantly. Remove from heat and add lemon juice, butter, and lemon zest. Pour into baked pie shell. Whip egg whites and cream of tartar to soft peaks. Gradually add sugar and beat to stiff peaks. Spread over filling, sealing to edges. Bake at 350° for 15-20 minutes until golden.

Yield: 1 9-inch pie

Puddings

Vanilla Pudding

- 3/4 c. sugar
- 5 T. ThickGel® or cornstarch
- ½ t. salt
- 3 c. milk
- 2 egg yolks
- ½ t. vanilla
- 2 T. butter or margarine

Combine sugar, cornstarch and salt in medium saucepan or double boiler. Add milk and stir until smooth. Cook over medium heat to a gentle boil, stirring constantly. Remove from heat. Stir egg yolks just until blended. Add a small amount of hot milk mixture to egg yolks, stirring constantly, then gradually add egg yolk mixture to hot mixture, stirring constantly. Return to a gentle boil and cook for 1 minute. Remove from heat and stir in vanilla and butter. Pour into a glass or plastic bowl and cover with plastic wrap or waxed paper, lightly touching the surface to prevent a skin from forming. Refrigerate.

Yield: 6 servings, filling for 12 cream puffs, or filling for 12 meringue shells

Cooked Pudding Variations

Chocolate Pudding: Prepare vanilla pudding as directed, mixing 1/4 cup cocoa into the dry ingredients before adding the milk. Increase butter to ¼ cup.

Coconut Cream Pudding: Prepare vanilla pudding as directed. When cool add 1 t. coconut extract. For pie filling add 2 c. flaked coconut and turn into a prepared pie shell.

Banana Pudding: Prepare vanilla pudding as directed. When cool add 1 t. banana flavoring. For pie filling, line pie shell with sliced bananas and top with banana pudding.

Instant Vanilla Pudding

- 2 c. cold milk
- 1/2 c. sugar
- dash salt
- 1/2 t. vanilla
- 2 drops yellow food coloring (opt.)
- 9-10 T. E-Z Gel®

Combine milk, sugar, salt, flavoring and coloring until sugar is dissolved. Gradually add E-Z Gel®, stirring with a wire whisk. Pudding will be soft set in 5 minutes.

Vanilla Custard

- 1 c. milk
- 1 c. cream
- 1/3 c. sugar
- ¼ t. salt
- 1 t. vanilla extract
- 2 eggs
- 2 egg yolks

Preheat oven to 350°. Combine milk and cream in microwave-safe bowl. Microwave on high for 2½ minutes until scalded. Stir in sugar, salt, and vanilla. Cool for five minutes. Whisk together eggs and egg yolks. Gradually whisk in the milk mixture, taking care not to incorporate air bubbles. Strain the custard through a wire mesh strainer lined with cheesecloth or heavy paper towel and divide into four custard cups.

Fold a kitchen towel to fit the bottom of a 9" x 13" cake pan and place the filled custard dishes in the pan. Place on middle rack of oven and add boiling water (1½ inches) in the space between the custard cups and the pan to form a water bath. Bake for 20-30 minutes until a knife inserted into the center comes out clean. Immediately remove from water bath and refrigerate before serving.

Yield: 4 servings

Crème Brûlée

Prepare Vanilla Custard as directed. Refrigerate to cool. Sprinkle each custard evenly with about 1 T. granulated sugar or coarse brown sugar. Method 1: Place on a baking sheet and broil, watching carefully to avoid burning, just until sugar melts to form a shiny glaze. Method 2: Quickly and evenly melt the sugar with a butane kitchen torch to make a smooth, even sheet of caramelized sugar.

Flan

Caramel:

- 1 c. sugar
- 1/3 c. water
- 2 T. light corn syrup

Custard:

- 1½ c. milk
- ½ c. whipping cream
- ½ c. sugar
- ¼ t. salt
- 1 t. vanilla extract
- 2 eggs
- 3 egg yolks

Preheat oven to 350°. Combine caramel ingredients in heavy frying pan over medium high heat. Stir until sugar is dissolved. Continue cooking until the sugar turns a light golden brown. Remove from heat and immediately pour into four custard cups, tilting to swirl caramel over bottom of each cup. Let set while preparing custard.

Combine milk and whipping cream in microwave-safe bowl. Heat in microwave for 2-2½ minutes until scalded. Stir in sugar, salt, and vanilla and cool for five minutes. Whisk together the eggs and egg yolks in medium bowl. Gradually whisk in the milk mixture, taking care not to incorporate air bubbles. Strain the custard through a wire mesh strainer lined with cheesecloth or heavy paper towels and divide into custard cups.

Fold a kitchen towel to fit the bottom of a 9" x 13" cake pan and place the filled custard dishes in the pan. Place on middle rack of oven and add boiling water (1½ inches) in the space between the custard cups and the pan to form a water bath. Bake for 20-30 minutes until a knife inserted into the center comes out clean. Immediately remove from water bath and refrigerate before serving. To unmold, run a knife gently around the edge of the custard cups and quickly invert onto plate.

Yield: 4 servings

Other Desserts and Sweet Sauces

Desserts

Dessert Crepes

- 2 eggs, lightly beaten
- ½ c. milk
- 1 T. melted butter
- ½ c. flour
- 1 T. sugar
- dash salt

Combine ingredients in blender container and blend for 1 minute. Lightly oil crepe pan or 8" sauté pan. Heat over medium high heat. Add ¼ c. batter to hot pan and swirl to coat. Cook until batter loses its shine. Turn and briefly cook other side if desired. Remove to platter and repeat with remaining batter. Fill baked crepes as desired.

Yield: 12 crepes

Cream Cheese Filling

- 3 oz. softened cream cheese
- ½ c. powdered sugar
- ½ c. whipping cream
- ½ t. vanilla

Beat together cream cheese and powdered sugar with electric mixer. Gradually add whipping cream and vanilla and beat until light and fluffy.

Yield: 1 cup

Sweet Sauces

Lemon Sauce

- 1 c. sugar
- 4 T. ThickGel® or cornstarch
- 2 c. water
- juice of one lemon

Combine sugar and cornstarch in small saucepan and stir to combine. Gradually add water and lemon juice and mix until well blended. Place over high heat, stirring constantly until mixture thickens. Reduce heat and boil for 1 minute. Cool slightly.

Yield: 2 cups

Vanilla Sauce

- ½ c. sugar
- 2 T. ThickGel® or cornstarch
- 1/4 t. salt
- 2 c. milk
- 2 drops yellow food color
- ½ t. vanilla
- 2 T. butter or margarine

Combine sugar, cornstarch and salt in medium saucepan or double boiler. Add milk and stir until smooth. Cook over medium heat to a gentle boil, stirring constantly. Remove from heat and fold in vanilla and butter.

Yield: 2-3 cups

Caramel Sauce

- 1/4 c. brown sugar
- 1/4 c. granulated sugar
- 3 T. ThickGel® or cornstarch
- 1/4 t. salt
- 2 c. milk
- ½ t. vanilla
- 2 T. butter

Combine sugars, cornstarch and salt in medium sauce pan or double boiler. Add milk and stir until smooth. Cook over medium heat to a gentle boil, stirring constantly. Remove from heat and fold in vanilla and butter.

Yield: 2-3 cups

Instant Fruit Glaze

- ½ c. sugar
- ½ t. fruit drink mix (Koolaid®)
- 1 c. water
- 4 T. E-Z Gel®
- 1½ c. sliced fruit, fresh or frozen

Combine sugar, fruit drink mix and water in a small bowl. Stir until dissolved. Gradually add E-Z Gel®, stirring constantly with wire whisk. Refrigerate 5 minutes to thicken. Fold in fresh or frozen fruit if desired. Serve over cake, ice cream, or other desserts. For fresh fruit pie filling, use 1/3 c. E-Z Gel. Fold in fresh fruit and turn immediately into prepared crust. Refrigerate before serving.

Yield: 2 cups fruit glaze

Fruit Glaze

- ½ c. sugar
- ½ t. fruit drink mix (Koolaid®)
- 2 T. cornstarch or ThickGel®
- 1 c. water
- 1½ c. sliced fruit, fresh or frozen

Combine sugar, fruit drink mix, and cornstarch in medium saucepan. Gradually add water until combined. Bring to a gentle boil over medium heat, stirring constantly. Simmer for three minutes until thick and bubbly. Remove from heat and cool for twenty minutes. Fold in fresh or frozen fruit. Serve over cake, ice cream, or other desserts. For fresh fruit pie filling, use 3 T. cornstarch or ThickGel®. Fold in fresh fruit and turn immediately into prepared crust. Refrigerate before serving.

Yield: 2 cups fruit glaze

E-Z Gel® Whipping Cream

- 1 pint whipping cream
- 1/2 c. powdered sugar
- 1 t. E-Z Gel®
- 1/2 t. vanilla

In a medium bowl, beat cream to form very soft peaks. Gradually add powdered sugar, EZ Gel and vanilla and whip to soft peaks. Store in refrigerator.

Hot Fudge Sauce

- 2 c. sugar
- 5 T. flour and 5 T. cocoa
- 1 12-oz can evaporated milk
- ¼ c. butter or margarine
- 1 t. vanilla

Combine sugar, flour, and cocoa in medium saucepan. Stir in evaporated milk and bring to boil. Reduce heat and simmer for 5-10 minutes, stirring constantly to desired thickness. Remove from heat and add butter and vanilla. Serve warm over ice cream or cake, or as the star in a banana split.

Yield: 16 servings

Note: This sauce thickens when standing. Add additional milk or cream to thin when reheating.

Simple Chocolate Sauce

- 1 pkg. semi-sweet chocolate chips
- 1/4 c. butter
- ½ c. evaporated milk or whipping cream
- 1 t. vanilla

Combine chocolate chips and butter in a medium saucepan. Heat until melted and smooth. Stir in milk or cream and heat until smooth. Do not boil. Remove from heat and add vanilla. Serve over ice cream, cake or pudding.

Yield: 1 ½ cups

Canning and Preserves

Basic Freezer Jam

- 3¾ c. crushed fruit (berries, peaches, etc.)
- 2 c. sugar
- ¼ c. lemon juice
- ½ c. E-Z Gel®

Combine fruit, sugar and lemon juice. Stir to dissolve sugar. Gradually add E-Z Gel®, stirring constantly. Let stand 5 minutes to thicken. Package, seal, label and freeze for 6-12 months.

Yield: 4½ cups

Cooked Apricot or Peach Jam

- 12 c. ground or chopped apricots or peaches
- 4 ½ c. sugar
- 2/3 c. ThickGel® do NOT substitute cornstarch
- 1 pkg. lemonade flavored drink mix (opt.)
- 3/4 c. lemon juice

Add 3 c. sugar to fruit and juice in heavy 6-8 quart pan. Bring to a boil over medium heat, stirring constantly. Combine remaining sugar and Thick Gel and stir into fruit mixture. Stir constantly until thick and bubbly. Add lemonade drink mix. Pour into sterilized pint jars, leaving 1/2" headspace. Adjust lids and process in water bath canner for 35 minutes.

Yield: about 7 pints

Apricot Barbecue Sauce

- 12 c. ground or chopped apricots
- 2 c. lime juice
- 6 c. sugar
- 1 1/3 c. ThickGel®
- 2 quarts catsup
- 30 whole allspice, crushed
- 40 whole cloves, crushed

Combine apricots and lime juice in heavy 6-8 quart pan. Stir in sugar and ThickGel® and bring to a boil, stirring constantly. Blend in remaining ingredients and boil for 1 minute. Fill jars, leaving 1/2" headspace. Adjust lids and process in water bath canner for 35 minutes (sea level).

Yield: 12 pints

Bottled Cherry Pie Filling

Utah State University Extension

- 6 quarts fresh or thawed sour cherries
- 7 c. sugar
- 1 ¾ c. ThickGel®
- 9 1/3 c. water or juice from cherries
- 2 t. almond extract (opt.)
- ½ c. bottled lemon juice
- 2 t. red food coloring (opt.)

Rinse and pit fresh cherries or thaw frozen cherries. Combine sugar and ThickGel® in large pot with water or juice from cherries. If desired, add almond extract and food coloring. Stir mixture and cook over medium heat until mixture thickens and begins to bubble. Add lemon juice and boil 1 minute, stirring constantly. Fold in cherries and fill jars with mixture, leaving ½" headspace. Adjust lids and process immediately in water bath canner for 30 minutes (sea level). Increase processing time for by 5 minutes for elevations of 1,000 to 3,000 feet and ten minutes for elevations from 3,000 to 5,000 feet.

Yield: 7 quarts

Bottled Apple Pie Filling

Utah State University Extension

- 6 quarts fresh apples, sliced ¼" thick
- 5 ½ c. sugar
- 1 ½ c. ThickGel®
- 1 T. cinnamon
- 1 t. nutmeg (opt.)
- 2 ½ c. cold water
- 5 c. apple juice
- ¾ c. bottled lemon juice

Peel, core and slice apples; place in water containing ascorbic acid. Blanch no more than 2 quarts at a time for 1 minute in boiling water and keep warm (See *Note).

Combine sugar, ThickGel® and spices in large pot with water, apple juice, lemon juice, and food coloring. Cook over medium heat until thick and bubbly. Fold in drained apple slices. Fill jars, leaving ½" head space. Adjust lids and process immediately in water bath canner for 35 minutes (sea level). Increase processing time for by 5 minutes for elevations of 1,000 to 3,000 feet and ten minutes for elevations from 3,000 to 5,000 feet.

Yield: 7 quarts

*Note: To blanch apple slices in the microwave, fill a 2-quart casserole dish full of loosely-packed apple slices and cover. Microwave just until apple slices change color and begin to lose their crispness (6-8 min.)

Bottled Blackberry Pie Filling

- 6 quarts fresh or thawed blackberries
- 5 ½ c. sugar
- 3 pkg. Raspberry Cranberry Koolaid® mix
- 2 c. ThickGel®
- 14 c. water
- ½ c. bottled lemon juice

Rinse fresh berries or thaw frozen berries. Combine sugar, Koolaid®, and ThickGel® in large pot with water. Stir mixture and cook over medium heat until mixture thickens and begins to bubble. Add lemon juice and boil 1 minute, stirring constantly. Fold in berries and fill jars with mixture, leaving ½" headspace. Adjust lids and process immediately in water bath canner for 30 minutes (sea level). Increase processing time for by 5 minutes for elevations of 1,000 to 3,000 feet and ten minutes for elevations from 3,000 to 5,000 feet

Yield: 7 quarts

Bottled Peach Pie Filling

- 6 qts. peeled sliced fresh peaches/apricots or nectarines
- 1 c. lemon juice
- water as needed
- 7 c. sugar
- 1 ½ c. ThickGel®
- 2 t. nutmeg (opt)

Combine peaches and lemon juice in large bowl. Sprinkle 3 cups sugar over peaches and let stand for 30 minutes. Drain accumulated juice. Reserve peaches and set aside. Add water to juice to equal 5 cups and place in a large heavy bottomed pan. Combine remaining sugar with ThickGel® and mix thoroughly. Add to juice and stir well. Bring to a boil over medium heat, stirring constantly. Stir in nutmeg. Fold in reserved peach slices and continue to cook until thick and bubbly. Immediately fill jars with mixture, leaving 1/2" headspace. Adjust lids and process immediately in water bath canner for 35 minutes (sea level).

Yield: 7 quarts

Canned Salsa

- 10 c. peeled, cored, chopped tomatoes (about 15)
- 6 c. seeded, chopped chili peppers* (2 lb.) Choose varieties for desired spiciness) OR 4 6½ oz. cans green chilies)
- 4 c. chopped onions (about 4)
- 1 6-oz. can tomato paste
- 3 t. salt
- ½ t. black pepper
- 1 c. vinegar (5%)
- 1/3 c. ThickGel®

Combine vegetables in large heavy saucepan. Add seasonings and tomato paste. Combine vinegar with ThickGel® and add to vegetables and stir until blended. Bring ingredients to a boil; simmer 10 minutes. Season to taste. Fill jars, leaving ½" headspace. Adjust lids and process in water bath canner for 30 minutes (sea level).

Yield: 6-8 pints

*Wear plastic gloves while preparing fresh peppers!

About the Author

Janet C. Stocks was raised on a small farm as the middlest of 7 children. She's been passionate about food for as long as she can remember. She has passed this love on to her six children, and anyone who has been fortunate enough to step foot into her kitchen or eat at her table. She started her first specialty food business in 1984 shortly after winning the Daily Herald cooking contest.

When her children were older, Janet returned to college and earned her BS and MS degrees from Brigham Young University in their Family Science department. Her masters degree centered on the benefits of families eating together and making meals in the home. She taught Meal Management and Household Equipment and developed new courses for Basic and Advanced Food Preparation. She taught at BYU for 12 years making amazing friends among the faculty and with her students.

While her formal teaching was a time she loved, Janet's food classes truly started with her six children, local youth groups, city and church groups, 4-H youth clubs, and so many others.

Janet and her brother, David, own and operate Cornaby's LLC, a growing food company that specializes in specialty cooking ingredients, bringing together all of their love for farm, food, and family.

Made in the USA
Monee, IL
04 November 2026

67380140R00125